THE
PSYCHIC
PSYCHOLOGIST®

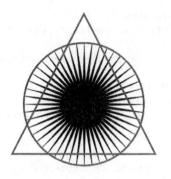

THE
PSYCHIC
PSYCHOLOGIST®

HEAL YOUR PAST
FIND PEACE IN THE PRESENT
TRANSFORM YOUR FUTURE

AMANDA CHARLES

HAY HOUSE

Carlsbad, California • New York City
London • Sydney • New Delhi

Published in the United Kingdom by:
Hay House UK Ltd, The Sixth Floor, Watson House, 54 Baker Street
London W1U 7BU
Tel: +44 (0)20 3927 7290; Fax: +44 (0)20 3927 7291; www.hayhouse.co.uk

Published in the United States of America by:
Hay House Inc., PO Box 5100, Carlsbad, CA 92018-5100
Tel: (1) 760 431 7695 or (800) 654 5126; Fax: (1) 760 431 6948 or (800) 650 5115
www.hayhouse.com

Published in Australia by:
Hay House Australia Ltd, 18/36 Ralph St, Alexandria NSW 2015
Tel: (61) 2 9669 4299; Fax: (61) 2 9669 4144; www.hayhouse.com.au

Published in India by:
Hay House Publishers India, Muskaan Complex, Plot No.3, B-2,
Vasant Kunj, New Delhi 110 070
Tel: (91) 11 4176 1620; Fax: (91) 11 4176 1630; www.hayhouse.co.in

A catalogue record for this book is available from the British Library.

Tradepaper ISBN: 978-1-78817-800-6
E-book ISBN: 978-1-78817-802-0
Audiobook ISBN: 978-1-78817-801-3

Interior images: Shutterstock

This product uses papers sourced from responsibly managed forests. For more
information, see www.hayhouse.co.uk

Printed and bound by CPI (UK) Ltd, Croydon CR0 4YY

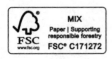

I hope this book touches your heart, in the same way that my heart was touched by those who died before I became the person with the wisdom to write it.

This book is to honour their lives.

It is to honour the lives of my two precious daughters, and all that they are.

It is to honour you, in your own life, and all you can become.

It is to honour my suffering, and the new life it called forth.

And it is to honour the process of living, fully connected, with the whole, authentic Self.

Embracing all of me...
hoping that you too can embrace all of you.

CONTENTS

LIST OF EXERCISES

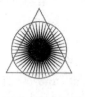

FOREWORD

For more than 35 years, I have answered so many questions about life after death and most things regarding the supernatural. On my journey, I had never come across anyone who challenged my understanding of such subjects or made me delve deeper into the furthest reaches of my mind to analyse my own beliefs – until I met Amanda Charles.

Amanda joined one of my teaching classes on developing mediumship at the College of Psychic Studies in London several years ago. Most of the students who attended these classes were already inclined to believe in an afterlife or had already had some sort of mediumistic experience which eased them onto the course. From the get-go, Amanda told me that despite having many experiences herself, she was still quite sceptical so would ask lots of questions, which I always encouraged. It didn't take me long to see that the type of question she posed was of a much deeper nature than the usual inquirer.

I wasn't sure if she would stay the course in the early days, as I believed that she might find it difficult to merge her more scientific, analytical belief system with her natural spiritual instinct. I needn't have been concerned as Amanda not only finished the course, but did so in the most triumphant way, showcasing her fantastic mediumship capability on stage for all to see. Hers was a great transformation; it had to be. To come from a background of psychology, with its forensic observations of behaviour and emotions, to a letting go and trusting a world unseen was truly a big ask, but the end result was a real breakthrough.

As a medium who has worked all over the world, I have come up against many psychologists, psychiatrists and other academics who have shown an interest in mediumship, but who kept enough distance as to remain on the fence of uncertainty. I always hoped that someone from this world would step up, look closer at the subject and bring a totally new perspective to the way we view human consciousness. The subject needs to be brought into the modern world and Amanda has absolutely done that with this wonderful book.

The Psychic Psychologist is a must for all who seek a better understanding of the human mind with all the trials and challenges it faces in this human experience. The book also brings a much clearer explanation regarding how spiritual growth can be born out of the experience of suffering, as well as providing the foundations to our healing when such growth is incorporated into our everyday lives.

What a pleasure to finally have such a great tool for spiritual advancement, which allows the reader to expand their higher consciousness while staying grounded in this reality. Great job, Amanda.

Gordon Smith
Internationally renowned medium, spiritual teacher and bestselling author

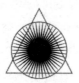

PREFACE

Sometimes we must trust in a new reality,
so that we may fully transform...

Have you ever had the privilege of watching a butterfly break free from the comfort of its chrysalis and engage with the struggles necessary for its survival? As a compassionate observer, it's so easy to feel compelled to help free this delicate damsel, yet it's this fight for freedom that marks the beginning of a distinctly new chapter in its life.

Its crypt-like cocoon, its own creation, was crafted as a safe space for progression, yet has simultaneously kept the caterpillar captive and bound. The new world of transformation that lies in wait is only unlocked through experiencing the very pain from which it may seek protection – a pain without which it may never fully develop, will most likely die, or will remain destined to live a life without flight.

Clueless to the bounty that lies ahead, it must surrender to the solitude, submerge itself in the suffering and allow the old reality to wither and die. But by letting go of the past and by trusting in the process of transformation, it remains open to new possibilities and to new perspectives as it soars up into the limitless sky.

Like the butterfly, this book shows me spreading my wings. It shows me shedding the skin of my former Self, surrendering suffering, eliminating illness and transforming my pain. Within its pages, I'm revealing my whole authentic Self and embracing all that is uniquely me. Like the caterpillar, I could have stayed in the darkness that engulfed me for so many years, leading a half-life, unable to see the full beauty that could emerge if I was to surrender to the process of change. Well, surrender I did. I chose to trust and to let go; no longer would I accept a life led by limitation.

So let me help *you* break out from your own self-imposed cocoon. Allow my words and my experiences to open your eyes to a *new* reality and guide you on your own journey of self-discovery and transformation, so that you too may take flight.

INTRODUCTION

My whole family is dead!

My mum, my brother, my father...

My sister-in-law, brother-in-law, father-in-law...

My grandparents, uncle, aunts...

All gone!

Dead!

Even my marriage is dead!

It could be suggested I know a few things about death, about suffering and about grief, and that would be true – I've encountered them all. There's that sudden disbelief stealing your breath as an unexpected dagger twists deep in your heart when a loved one is snatched away in an instant. Then there's that long, laboured death, the kind that took my dad for example, creeping in over a decade, his body betraying him through a gradual paralysis, leaving his mind untouched, yet there he remained – trapped, locked in, alone. There's that all too familiar death from those twisted vines of cancer suffocating the soul until nothing but a mere skeleton remains. Even that present but absent kind of death that leaves the physical body intact while fading out the personality, until it's all but a forgotten memory – the person you once knew, long since gone.

That's the harsh reality of life. No matter who you are, no matter what you do, no matter how poor or great your circumstances, your health or your wealth, the universal truth of life is that in one way or another, death is ever-present.

Some of you will be connecting with these words, remembering painful losses you've encountered in your *own* life, whereas others will not. But for all of us, death comes with many faces; it's not only there in the vacant chairs around the dinner table, it's in the emptiness that echoes from the walls of our home when it's time to move on, it's in our relationships once the love is lacking and the excitement has long since expired, and it's in that dread rising in our stomach when that longed-for occupation has diminished to mere obligation.

To talk of death, loss and the permanency of endings outside the therapy room is often seen to be taboo. As a society, we'd rather dismiss the depth of feeling and discomfort that comes alongside such finality. Yet we will all swallow our own dose of suffering at one time or another, in whatever form it takes, and when doing so, can choose to embrace it as an amazing opportunity for growth, for healing and for transformation. It's through experiencing and accepting the death of what once was, and releasing the inevitable aftermath, that we can embrace a process of change and healing so that life can be birthed anew. That's what this book is about.

It has come not only from my clinical but from my lived experience. The sudden loss of those I loved is merely one example of the long and painful encounters with life's lessons that have led me to share this process with you today. It was tragedy and illness that forced me to acknowledge how disconnected I was from my Self and begin the process of reconnection at every level of my existence – body, heart, mind and soul. It's from this pool of suffering and wealth of wisdom that this book has been birthed, in the hope that I may help prevent *you* from suffering in the same way that I had to, or at the very least open the doorway to new possibility.

Today, many people call me 'The Psychic Psychologist', a label I've struggled to wear, having valiantly fought the exposure of my psychic side for many years. But, just like every worthy opponent, each and every time I knocked it down, it came back stronger, eventually leaving me with no other move than to simply surrender.

I remember its origins well. I squirmed the first time Gordon Smith, hailed as the UK's most accurate medium, identified me as such. In my mind, I mocked. As if I, a respected and successful chartered counselling psychologist, with my work contingent upon and defined by science, would *ever* allow myself to be associated with such an unsubstantiated field marred by stigma and controversy! As if I would *ever* endorse the exposure of this precarious part of my life. What would my clients say? My colleagues? My peers?

After all, the word 'psychic' is such a loaded term, and aligning myself with its use professionally felt like setting myself up as a target for people to take aim at with their arrows laced with negative judgement and fixed opinion. The truth is, it's taken many significant events for me to accept and honour what some have described as my 'gifts', including repeatedly predicting the future by seeing down timelines and having precognitive dreams, sensing illness in others, facilitating my own healing and that of others, and experiencing after-death communication, spontaneous transfiguration, astral projection, spiritual channelling and inter-dimensional travel.

I have always been more than aware that claims of such occurrences are open to allegations of falsehood or fantasy, due to a lack of scientific validation. As a scientist myself, with my clinical work and research grounded in evidence-based practice, it's been a great challenge to accept this other world, one that consists of phenomena that cannot be easily measured or robustly replicated.

It was this inner conflict that led me to Gordon. It was 2004, my mum had just died and she'd been repeatedly making contact with me. I would see her, feel her and hear her, but was constantly questioning whether this after-death communication (ADC) was merely 'magical thinking' – a misinterpretation of sensory experiences often associated with the supernatural, *especially* after the loss of a loved one. I had always looked for scientific explanations for the paranormal phenomena I'd experienced, but much of my mum's contact couldn't be explained away scientifically – like when she was directing me to things that were needed for her funeral. Things like her address book, which was *always* kept in the same place, yet was nowhere to be found until she told me it was in the glove compartment of my dad's car. Even the location of a necklace my dad wanted her to wear for the funeral was projected into my mind as an image, revealing it was wrapped up in a sealed box at my mother-in-law's house. I had no prior knowledge of this box, had no idea why the necklace wasn't with the rest of my mum's jewellery, and most certainly didn't expect it to be at my in-laws' – until I checked, and there it was!

I was crying out to know for certain whether this contact was real. Do we *really* survive death, or was this just fantasy? I asked to be shown something that couldn't be disputed, and no sooner had the thought entered my mind than I felt compelled to switch on the TV. There was a BBC2 documentary following Gordon Smith as he gave a mediumship reading to a couple who had lost their son. Gordon's accuracy was clearly evident, but I wasn't to be fooled – it was a TV programme, after all!

But then, 'He will show you beyond all reasonable doubt,' said a voice in my mind I knew was not my own.

That sentence marked the beginning of my journey. Fast-forward to the following year and I was sitting in the audience at a Gordon Smith event with thousands of other people hoping to hear from those they had loved and lost. This was my first encounter with mediumship. Friends had bought me the ticket for my 30th birthday, as I felt confident the voice had meant a reading from Gordon would settle my conflicting thoughts once and for all. Sadly, I left the hall feeling deflated, as there had been no message for me – this was not where I would leave my doubts behind.

Yet the voice had brought with it such certainty that I decided to queue for the book signing to ask Gordon personally how I could arrange a reading.

To cut a long story short, he was no longer offering readings, and I haven't had a reading from him in the 18 years since, yet the voice was still correct. Through Gordon, I have indeed been shown, *beyond all reasonable doubt*, the answer to my question; it just wasn't in the way I *expected* to see it. Instead, it was in the way I *needed* to see it – through my *own* lived experience!

Instead of seeking guidance, direction and answers from outside myself, I attended numerous trainings with Gordon. Initially, I was on a mission to expose the 'paranormal' events I'd experienced throughout my life as the mere workings of an elaborate imagination, misinterpretations, coincidences or even flukes. In fact, the joke was on me, as the process brought forth a surprising realization of the magnitude of the metaphysical and the opportunities it held for the enhancement of our mental, physical, emotional and relational health and wellbeing.

What I needed, I already possessed, and had I not realized this, I'd have been dependent on Gordon, or someone like him, to provide me with something I was actually able to do for myself. This is one of the reasons why I now choose to combine the psychic and the psychologist rather than offering mediumship or psychic readings. This life lesson, amongst many others, has shown me the value of empowering people to connect with all their levels of Self and to develop their *own* inner guidance and healing, rather than give away their power and autonomy to someone else.

I wasn't always comfortable with this, however. I remember the first time a 'sixth sense' unwittingly infiltrated a client session. I'd only been in private practice for a short while, but my connection with this particular client had been off the scale from the very beginning. She was a young professional dancer with two small children, and having felt 'a bit depressed and unsatisfied' in recent months, she felt she needed a little help to find herself once more.

From the moment we first met, I just seemed to know everything she was going to say before she said it – I mean *literally* word for word. Now, this could have been down to a deeply empathic connection, but it was much more than that. Somehow, without being told, I even knew of events that had occurred in her life during the week since our previous session.

I would reflect back and interpret her words using metaphorical language, as I did with many other clients, but I was always met with responses like 'You've just described the exact image I'm seeing in my mind' or 'Are you psychic or something?!'

Then the moment came when I could hide no more.

'I walked into this bookshop,' she said excitedly, 'and this book stood out to me. I just had to buy it, and it's changed my life!'

'Barbara Brennan, *Hands of Light*,' I responded.

To this day, I have no idea how those words left my mouth – it seemed to happen at a level beyond reason, beyond reflection and beyond thought.

A horrified look filled her face. 'How on earth did you know that?' she asked. 'Of all the books in all the world, how did you know it was that exact book I bought?'

There was no answer I could give that could explain away how the image of that specific book cover had flashed in front of my eyes. I couldn't even suggest it was a lucky guess, as it bore no relevance to her life. I could do nothing to appease her confusion, and despite brushing the discomfort away with a joke, I think deep down, neither of us could recover from what those few words had meant – there's being seen as a client, and there's *really* being seen! Our sessions ended a few weeks later.

Perhaps this experience so early on in my career contributed to how guarded I became around bringing these two worlds together. My journey to doing so consisted of two approaches: one in total denial, masquerading as the paranormal police and only accepting that which could be considered concrete, and the other discreetly exploring the intangible and gathering more and more evidence of its existence.

My work remains, however, grounded in science, just like that of every other psychologist, but, having done extensive research to find a scientific basis to support the more intuitive aspect of my work, I now also incorporate the field of quantum physics – the science that prompted the leaps in technology that enabled the development of the internet, smart phones, MRI scanners, GPS and LED lights. Through observing the surprising behaviour of sub-atomic particles, scientists discovered that everything was interconnected. Despite appearances, we're not separate solid physical objects; at a sub-atomic level, we consist of waves of energy with their own vibrational frequency. It's this energetic field that we can use to facilitate positive and lasting change in our lives. We have a physical body and an emotional body, but we also have an energy body, so by incorporating quantum physics, we gain the scientific validity to support working with both the physical and the metaphysical.

This grounding in quantum physics is one of the main elements that makes my proficiency as a psychologist different from most. Psychologists are not routinely taught about quantum physics, or usually aware of the energy body, but focus mainly on identifying maladaptive thoughts, feelings and behaviours, the key experiences that have facilitated their development, and how these patterns impact the Self and others. Armed with this information, they may then look to diagnose and 'treat' the resulting 'disorders'. Yet without acknowledging or addressing the *energetic* element of the Self, they can often find treatment outcomes very limited and short-lived. In my experience, the energetic is the very realm through which our difficulties are made manifest, so it's for this reason that I incorporate this element in my practice and it's why it features so prominently throughout this book. If we can only see a part of the problem, then we're also blind to a part of the solution, and the energetic realm is the missing link that must be addressed.

In addition, my work draws on research in the fields of epigenetics (the interaction between genes and the environment), psycho-neuro-immunology (the intricate links between mind, body and immune function) and psycho-neuro-endocrinology (the interplay between psychological processes and the hormonal system). This promotes both an evidence-based consideration and an open and objective awareness of the amazing opportunities that exist for us when we consciously step away from living life on autopilot.

Through sharing my knowledge and experience with you, my hope is that you may awaken within you an awareness of a new reality, one where you can embrace your own authentic Self and live as a multi-dimensional being, sparing yourself that dose of despair dispensed by a 'life-school' that teaches through a syllabus of turmoil and pain. Equally, if that boat to breakdown has already set sail, my hope is that these words will reach you, provide some light in your darkness and inspire the necessary actions to steer you to a more favourable destination.

You don't need to wait for disaster to descend before setting transformation in motion, however. By engaging with this book, you'll gain the knowledge and skills to construct a fulfilling future of your own conscious choosing.

Of course, you may have picked up this book because you've already endured some terribly traumatic experiences. Some of you will be gasping for air, drowning in the present moment as the tides of trauma pull you under, whilst others will be basking in the safety of dry land, unaware of that future tsunami waiting to engulf and overshadow the person they are yet to become. Wherever you find yourself, know that I have walked the path from trauma to transformation and I am walking alongside you throughout this book, my personal insights and professional experience sketching out the process through which you can turn your pain into progress and take the highway to happiness rather than the road to ruin.

What I'd like to bring to your conscious awareness is how much of your suffering in the present, *regardless* of how it's expressed – through panic, obsession or addiction, for example – grows from, and is formed within the same roots – roots from the past left unattended and abandoned through a disconnect from, or denial of, a fully integrated and authentic Self.

This is your opportunity to connect with that Self – to connect with who you are at all levels of your existence – and to call in who you wish to become. You have *everything* you need within you to realize your full potential, and with the combined wisdom of your intuitive-Self and your future-Self for guidance, the opportunities for transformation really are endless.

Wherever you are in your life right now, you get to choose how to live it day by day, moment by moment, decision by decision. As such, you always have the most amazing opportunity available to you – which is that you can begin again. When you realize you aren't on the right path, you get to begin again; when you find you're repeating dysfunctional patterns from the past, you get to begin again; and when you fall off the wagon, or make a mistake, *again*, you get to pause, take a deep breath and begin again once more. In each and every moment you get to assess whether a particular decision, thought, emotion or behaviour takes you one step closer to becoming the future-Self you desire, whether it keeps you trapped in the now, or whether it pulls you back into reinstating past pain, taking you further away from connecting with the person you've always had the innate potential to become.

So, this is not a book about grief, about death, or about divorce; this is a book about *living*. It's about connecting with each and every layer of your existence to free yourself from suffering, transform your pain, go beyond your limitations and generate that life you'd love to live. It's a book that will help you tap more deeply into your higher power and follow your inner voice, so you can transform your reality and consciously construct positive change in your present and for your future. So, no matter how many times life has kicked you when you're down, and no matter what difficulties you are dealing with as a result, this book will show you, it will *prove* to you, that when you are fully connected on all levels of the Self you *can* break free from your past, transform your trauma, process your pain and learn to live a life you love.

THE PROCESS EXPLAINED

I can't begin to know what journey you have been on and I can't begin to see the impact of what you're carrying as a result, but what I do know and what I can do is to tell you *my* truth, in the hope that this connects you to your *own*. Throughout this book you'll hear stories from my own personal life experience and you'll hear professional anecdotes from my client work, and even discover some findings from scientific research, but most importantly, you'll begin to hear your own inner guidance and open your heart and mind to the infinite possibilities you hold inside.

To facilitate this, the book is split into two parts: Part I, An Awareness of Self, and Part II, The Connected Self. Part I provides the foundational work for you to gain an understanding and awareness of the Self and the repercussions of disconnection from it. You can also explore your own current Self-connection through a quiz that will reveal which levels of Self you're likely to be disconnected from or over-identified with and where you're needing more healing and balance.

Part II focuses on that healing and balance, on generating a fully Connected Self, using my Release and Re-programming Method. It takes you through a gradual process of reconnection on all levels of the Self and across all of time. First, you'll connect with the 'present-past' by travelling back down your timeline to learn how and why events before, during and after your birth may be having a detrimental impact on your life in the now. From here, you'll understand how and why you've become the person you are today, and it will bring into your conscious awareness what conditioning from that past is being unconsciously projected onto your present and your future. Then you'll move to connecting with your present-Self and employ strategies to generate a peaceful present, enabling you to switch off your stress-response system so you can move on to safely processing any pain from your past and removing the blocks and conditioning that can inhibit your future growth. You'll do this at each level of the Self – physically, emotionally, mentally and spiritually – by following my Hierarchy of Healing protocol. Then you'll connect with your future-Self timeline and embed this programming in the present, consciously calling this new reality into your life.

This process brings together traditional psychological interventions, energy work and healing practices, and can be applied as effectively to healing a health crisis as to challenging self-destructive behaviour patterns, walking away from the wrath of the workplace and righting repeated wrongdoings in relationships.

For some of you, it may be wise to enlist a therapist as you take this journey, especially if you have a strong history of mental illness or multiple traumas in your past. Others may choose to do so just for the additional one-to-one support, or to gain help with those blind spots we all have and may struggle to become aware of. Either way, remember *you* are the expert on you, and a part of the premise of this book is to show that when fully connected to your whole, authentic Self, you can be your own best healer!

Change can be scary, of course, and letting go of the known can be tough – even if it is what you're wanting. So, be gentle with yourself, and start, if you wish, by just showing up and engaging with this book each day, even if just for 20 minutes. Allow yourself the gift of curiosity and openness as you connect with the teachings. The act of repeatedly choosing your own wellbeing over and above any competing demands sends out the important vibration of intention and calls in positive change – effortlessly. In time, this choice gets wired into your behaviour and your brain, and then the magic can't *not* happen! This simple action will ignite your energy, swell your self-regard and orchestrate an outlook that can only bring more clarity to all you wish to become. So, have a look at your schedule and make a regular slot each day *just* for this – *just* for *you*.

After all, this book is for you.

If you feel burnt-out and exhausted every day, have a chronic illness that affects the quality of your life, or even feel your life looks perfect from the outside but on the inside you're secretly falling apart, this book is for you.

If you've gone from one practitioner to the next, tried numerous treatments in the hope that *this will be the one that works* and yet still you suffer, this book is for you.

If you're wanting to make *any* kind of change in your life, this book is for you.

It's for your friends.

It's for your family.

It's for your future!

So, what are you waiting for? All you need is a journal to keep track of your progress.

Ready now? Let's dive in. Let's do the work to help you to help yourself.

RESOURCES

The exercises included in this book are also available to download from my website, along with worksheets, audio tracks and other bonus material. Visit **thepsychicpsychologist.com/book-resources**. The audio tracks can also be found in the audiobook, which is available in the *Empower You Unlimited Audio* app or wherever you listen to your audiobooks.

PART I

AN AWARENESS
OF SELF

CHAPTER 1

THE SELF

What do I mean by the Self exactly, and what does it mean to be fully connected? As you may not be familiar with these terms, it feels important to define exactly what I'm referring to, so we can share the same understanding.

DEFINITIONS

In the field of psychology, the numerous definitions of what constitutes the Self can leave people a little confused. Many differing schools of thought are competing to promote their 'truth', based on the specific characteristics that underpin each theoretical orientation. But regardless of origins, the Self is a complex, multi-faceted construct that plays a fundamental role in shaping human behaviour, motivation and wellbeing.

The concept of Self-connection is relatively new, and there's limited scientific research to draw upon. A recent study by Klussman and colleagues[1] defines it as a subjective experience consisting of three interrelated components: self-awareness, self-acceptance and self-alignment.

- **Self-awareness:** A noticing of one's internal experience – thoughts, emotions, sensations, preferences, values, resources and intuition.

- **Self-acceptance:** Having an openness to oneself and fully acknowledging and supporting, without judgment, those relevant characteristics and experiences held as belonging to who you are.

- **Self-alignment:** Using self-knowledge to behave in ways that are consistent with, and authentically reflect, one's internal states, preferences, resources and intuitions.

To have Self-connection requires all three components, effectively meaning we're authentically acting in alignment with our awareness of the Self, from a place of non-judgement and Self-acceptance.

Whilst I agree with this definition, which was born from and validated through this research, as The Psychic Psychologist®, I feel the need to expand it a little.

As we grow, interact and explore in childhood, we begin to form a mental image, or template, of who we believe we are, of who we believe others to be, and of our place in and relationship with the world around us. So, as an adult, when asked who we think we are, we'll most likely draw upon these earlier impressions. This is our identity, it's how we identify ourselves to others and to ourselves, and it will most likely include our physical attributes, inner character and emotional temperament, and probably some kind of autobiographical narrative. Perhaps we identify as a loser in love, for example, having never found that *one* soul to light up our life, or maybe we associate ourselves with success, having achieved everything we've set our sights on.

This Self we identify with most often refers to the internalized conditioning that's repeatedly wired into our brain, yet in focusing on what we *do* (or have done), we fail to recognize the true essence of who we *really are*. You see, we *can* be all of this, yet we are simultaneously much, much more, and it's this intangible element I also refer to when talking of the Self.

THE INTANGIBLE SELF

This is that unique Self that lives within each and every one of us and is more a state of *being* than a state of *doing*. It's who we are when all the labels have been stripped away. We're not our job, our disease or our role as a parent or child, we're the constant that lies within – a conscious awareness, an intangible, unchanging, energetic *presence*, regardless of how we identify at any one time.

Interestingly, the field of quantum physics recognizes this invisible realm, and some scientists put this forward as evidence that not only does this energy exist, but it's the sole governing influence over matter, guiding the behaviour of particles and shaping reality.[2,3]

In brief, quantum physics is a branch of science that investigates the laws of nature at the microscopic level. Everything in the physical world, including inanimate objects, is made up of tiny units called atoms. Quantum physics has revealed these aren't solid particles, as was once believed, they just look solid because the electrons spin around the nucleus so very fast. They are in fact suggested to be mostly empty space – 99.99 per cent empty space to be precise.[4] Just think about that for a moment. This means that 99.99 per cent of everything you can see and touch isn't actually solid, it's just vibrating energy – and that includes us!

This empty space exists mainly between the positively charged nucleus of the atom and the negatively charged electrons that orbit around it, emitting waves of light energy at different frequencies as they move between energy levels or interact with other particles. This means that everything in the Universe, seen and unseen, is in its very essence a *wave of energy* with its own unique vibrational frequency and speed. Even when matter appears to be completely inert and solid, such as the laptop on which I'm typing these words, it is composed of sub-atomic particles whizzing around in a perpetual state of motion. As such, all things, great and small, have their own energy, which influences the energetic environment around us and within us!

Please hold this in mind as I touch upon the perspective of Self given by cell biologist Dr Bruce Lipton. Decades of studying stem cells led him to subscribe to the view that we're far more than our physicality. He proposes that cell membranes function as information processors with tiny antennas responding to a field of energy and suggests that we receive a unique 'broadcast signal' correlating to our individual vibrational frequency. Each person's antennas, referred to as Self-receptors, can only receive their specific information, enabling their body to know what's Self and what's not. So, as we're all biologically different, if we take an organ from one person and transplant it into another, the immune system flags it up as 'non-Self' and looks to eliminate it. This is why transplant patients typically receive immunosuppressant drugs to reduce the risk of organ rejection.

This could also be one potential factor behind how, despite the constant regeneration and replacement of cells within our body, our physical complaints remain. Psychological, lifestyle and environmental factors play a part, but we must also consider the possibility that it's because our energetic frequency identifies us as that suffering Self.

So, whilst we may have been conditioned to think of the Self as our mind or our physical body, this theory potentially supports the more spiritual view that our body is just the *receiver* of who we are and the vehicle for its expression.

THE SELF AS CONSCIOUSNESS – AN ENERGETIC BROADCAST SIGNAL

So, could it be that the Self is the specific broadcast frequency of energy/ consciousness that is received by the body and mind and projected out into the world as who we are? In the same way that our favourite broadcast show is neither the actual TV set nor the radio, perhaps we're more than our physical body and maybe we're not within our mind.

Interestingly, this theory makes sense of how the Self can persist even in the absence of normal brain functioning, and how some people with brain damage can still perceive correctly. For example, some individuals with damage to the visual cortex are still able to perceive visually.[5] Perhaps what's damaged is just a part of the physical interface receiving the signal, whilst the transmission of frequency/consciousness remains intact, and in some circumstances, finds a new connection within the physical receiver or helps repair the old. The brain may be compensating for the damage by reorganizing its functions or repairing or rerouting to new pathways, but what's governing that? Could it be that it's the consciousness itself that is restructuring the brain? Or perhaps it's that we actually perceive through *consciousness* and not through the physical structures of the brain at all. These points are all up for debate, and are presented here to remind us all to keep an open mind.

THE LEVELS OF THE SELF

My personal philosophy is that the Self is multi-dimensional. That we exist in a space of dense, low-vibrating physiological form, from which we interact with the physical world, yet simultaneously we have a biochemical dimension to us, an element of thought, an emotional field and a higher, faster vibrational field of consciousness. I believe this is how we are able to create from the level of conscious thought and bring that into physical reality – but only once we align that reality on all the energetic levels of the Self.

I see the levels of the Self as being analogous to ice, water and steam, where the chemical composition is the same (H_2O), but they have different vibrational frequencies, molecular arrangements and physical properties. The physical body is solid and dense, with tightly packed molecules vibrating at a low frequency, like ice. The emotions, with their higher-vibrational frequency, are like water, with its freely moving, fluid molecules that change form. Then there are the realms of thought and spirit, with their intangible and expansive form, which can be compared to the gaseous state of steam, moving at a higher, faster frequency than a solid or liquid. I believe that we exist on all these levels at the same time and that they are all interconnected, which is why we must address our healing on all of them.

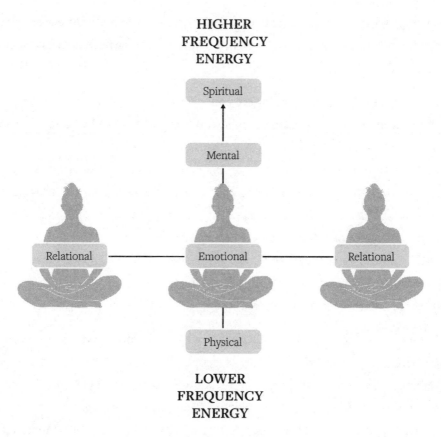

HIGHER
FREQUENCY
ENERGY

Spiritual

Mental

Relational — Emotional — Relational

Physical

LOWER
FREQUENCY
ENERGY

The Energetic Levels of Self

To illustrate this interconnectedness, let's take an experience you may have had as a child, when perhaps your teacher humiliated you in front of the class, or your friends shamed you because of your appearance, culture, class or race. Whilst you were likely to be very aware of how that made you feel, it didn't *only* impact you on an emotional level. Yes, you felt embarrassment, shame, anger, perhaps even fear, but that distress was expressed through all the other levels of the Self too, whether you were consciously aware of it or not.

All of those emotions are biochemical messengers, and are felt as sensations in the body – flushed face, muscular tension, sweating, increased heart rate, etc. As there is a perceived threat, the stress-response system is activated too, so alongside the biochemical cocktail of emotions, the body is flooded with the impact of this stress, and remains vulnerable to the physical disorders that can be triggered as a result.

On a mental level, this situation can provoke a whole host of negative thinking about yourself, other people and the world around you. It can lead to limiting beliefs about your capabilities and distorted thinking patterns; perhaps you become overly critical, believing you're inadequate or flawed, maybe you start overgeneralizing this situation and applying it to others, or start catastrophizing or exaggerating the negative consequences of the humiliating event. It can have long-lasting effects on your relationship with yourself, decreasing self-esteem and confidence, and can prompt or exacerbate a bout of anxiety, depression, or numerous other mental health disorders and physical conditions.

The impact of this event can also permeate your relationships with others. Perhaps you become mistrustful, as people no longer seem predictable or safe, so you withdraw and avoid situations where you might possibly become humiliated further, judged or rejected. If you also struggle with feelings of inadequacy or social anxiety, it might extend beyond this, impacting your ability to form new relationships, connect with others or engage in social situations.

The influence it might have on a spiritual level can vary, based on your individual beliefs and values, but if you've been left feeling inadequate or unworthy, you might lose faith in yourself and others, which can translate to losing faith in and connection with a higher power and purpose, hindering your spiritual development and zest for life.

So, can you see how we can become the conduit through which these unconscious programmes from past predicaments (even just one challenging encounter) play out in the present day? Such experiences merge into our sense of Self, the repercussions of which invariably play out through our actions, our emotions and our thoughts, infiltrating our expectations of ourselves and others. We're inadvertently left to walk a predestined path that's built upon the unprocessed difficulties of our past, which become projected onto our present and thus play out in our future.

Without intervention, this keeps us trapped at that same energetic frequency, bound for more of what came before and chained to a world of dysfunction, disability, discontentment and even disease. There is an idea, often attributed to Einstein, that a problem cannot be solved from the same level of consciousness that created it. If this is true, to shift our perspective and the fortunes of our future, we must first connect with our whole Self at a higher, wiser level of functioning. In my experience, not only do the levels of the Self move up from dense to lighter consciousness, but as well as having a physical body, we also have an energy body that mirrors the physical – and it is here that this higher Self resides.

Physical Self	Energetic Self
Physical body	Energy body
Emotion	Heart consciousness
Thinking mind	Higher mind
Observing mind	Individual consciousness
Relationship with others	Collective consciousness

More research is required before we can fully understand the relationship between consciousness and the levels of the Self. To explore this concept further, let's consider a client of mine with a condition called dissociative identity disorder (DID).

The Many Selves of 'Grace'

Previously known as multiple personality disorder, dissociative identity disorder is a complex psychological condition involving an extreme form of disconnection from the consciousness of the physical Self, where a person's thoughts, memories, feelings, actions and even identity can become lost, at least for a time. Alongside this is the existence of a minimum of two distinct personality states or 'identities', described as alternate personalities or 'alters', that present as totally separate individuals.

It has long been suggested that this dissociative aspect is a coping mechanism that shuts awareness off from that which is too painful to assimilate into the conscious Self. This has been proposed because as many as 99 per cent of individuals who go on to develop DID have a history of life-threatening traumas or abuse during childhood.[6] People like my client 'Grace',* for example, who to the outside world looks and breathes as Grace, while inside it may be hours, even days, since the Self as *she* knows it was last present. During this interlude, Grace is 'offline' and a different Self, or number of Selves, take centre stage. When Grace comes back 'online', she'll often 'wake up' in hospital, recovering from physical harm, unaware of the devastation and destruction that have occurred in her absence.

In my experience, this is more than the switching off of reality due to a defence mechanism, and unlike some budding actress switching to a different identity from her extensive repertoire, Grace actually switches to different Selves. When they appear, where does she go? How come she has absolutely no awareness of herself or of other people present during this time, and how does this process actually occur?

These are questions traditional psychology just can't answer. But what if we were to tentatively consider applying Dr Bruce Lipton's theory: that our Self-receptors receive a broadcast that we then identify as the Self? What

---

* Names have been changed to maintain confidentiality.

if the involuntary Self-switching in DID is more than a coping mechanism triggered as protection from an unspeakable reality? What if it is occurring at the energetic level of the Self?

The chapters that follow provide evidence that trauma changes the biochemistry of the body and can alter the physiology and the expression of the genes, so what if acute or chronic trauma during the developmental stages of childhood impacts the biology or physiology of the cell membrane – the antenna – and thus its capacity to receive the constant stream of a single Self? Perhaps we can adapt to a traumatic environment to such a degree that we can alter our Self-receptors – tuning in to new frequencies, switching them on and off, or even shutting them down for a while. The Self might simply go offline, allowing the consciousness of a new frequency to be online for a time.

DID research has already shown different physiology from one Self to another. When a new Self is present, they not only bring with them their own thought processes and habitual feelings, their own personal preferences and characteristics, but most significantly, their own physiology, to the extent that one Self can be diagnosed with a particular medical condition and yet in the others there's no evidence of it. Researchers have revealed blindness and deafness in one alter, yet not in others,[7] and some alters with allergic reactions, yet others without.[8] In fact, a study by Frank Putnam, Professor of Psychiatry at the University of North Carolina, found 26 per cent of 100 patients with DID experienced different allergies across personality states.[9] In the same study, Putnam noted that 37 per cent of his patients also had different dominant writing hands amongst personalities, a finding also noted elsewhere, alongside changes in handwriting script.[10,11]

Other notable differences in the various personality states of DID participants as compared to single personality controls include blood pressure,[12] response to medication, autonomic, immune and endocrine function,[13] and visual functioning.[14] One person was even diagnosed with full blindness following craniocerebral trauma and gradually regained her sight in her other personalities.[15]

These research findings provide evidence to suggest that people can literally have a different body when presenting as a different personality. Pharmacologist and neuropsychiatrist Dr Candace Pert suggested that this is evidence that consciousness creates reality. At the very least, it suggests that our body can change depending on what state of mind we're in.

This makes me ponder where physical issues are stored. How can they reside locally in the body when the body can be so different with a simple shift in personality or consciousness? Perhaps the imprint of an illness that relates to an identity is first stored within the frequency of the Self and not specifically within the DNA body. Epigenetics has shown that it's actually the environment that switches a gene on or off; in a similar way, perhaps it's the external broadcast of consciousness that programmes the body. This relates well to energy healing, in particular distance healing, as here we're effectively retuning the frequency and thus the information received by the body.

'Grace' – the Evidence

For many years it was a mammoth task for Grace to gain appropriate treatment from the medical profession, as many consultants refused to accept the validity of her DID diagnosis. Amazingly, however, when she 'switched' to her seven-year-old alter 'Lily' during a QEEG brain-mapping analysis, the resulting change in brain imagery validated the separate Selves within. It also called into question who we are as 'the Self'.

Conventional biology would have you believe it's physical proteins and DNA that make you who you are, yet the moment Grace switched to a different Self, with her separate identity, preferences, beliefs, values, even age, her brain altered with it. No longer was the pattern of Grace's brain-mapping visible; within seconds, as she stepped back, a new brain was revealed – a less mature and more disorganized brain, reflecting the specific Self that was seven-year-old Lily. This new brain imagery showed brainwave frequencies consistent with the brain of a young child, along with patterns of psychiatric conditions, personality traits and developmental issues very different from those seen in the images moments before. Interestingly, the characteristics observed totally related to how people experienced Lily, and were in no way relevant to how Grace presented.

The way Grace describes connecting with her alters and consciously facilitating the switching process is also fascinating to me, as it's very similar to how I connect with the energetic frequency of another person – either through mediumship, if they have no physical body, or through a psychic connection, if they do. The term I have personally coined for both these connections is 'telempathy', as for me, regardless of whether a person is dead or alive, it's the same process – I'm merging with their energetic frequency via an empathic and telepathic connection.

Grace had been unsure if switching during the QEEG was possible, so throughout the day she had spoken of how exciting it would be if a younger part came through, hoping they were listening and would be intrigued enough to come forward. When the moment arrived, she deliberately retreated in her mind, leaving space for whoever was to appear – the same process used by mediums when stepping aside to allow 'overshadowing' by another consciousness.

Now, I'm not making any specific claims here, I'm simply noting with curiosity some similarities between two very different fields of experience that may warrant further contemplation, as such findings call into question who we are as an individual Self. If we can switch to a different Self within our own body, with distinct personalities and brain patterns and potentially varied chemistry, biology and physiology, it challenges the notion of a fixed physical Self. From this perspective we could conclude that it's the consciousness of the Self that informs our body about our identity, not the other way around.

If true, this bolsters the possibilities for conscious Self-transformation through actively changing the frequency of our energy, alongside adapting our thoughts, feelings and behaviours – a process we'll explore later in this book.

THE CONNECTED SELF

So, when viewing the Self through the lens of quantum science, we're not just a solid, physical human *doing*, we're concurrently an energetic human *being*. Therefore, when fully connected with the Self, you'll be in touch with, and fully conscious of, all that you are on every level – physical, emotional, mental, spiritual and relational. As you gain alignment on all these levels, and act accordingly, you can activate your own inner guidance and tap into your own innate capacity for Self-healing and Self-fulfilment. In doing so, you can become the master of your own destiny rather than seeking solace and direction from somewhere outside yourself, opening the door to better health, better healing and a better, more authentic life.

Preparing to Reconnect

To prepare for this journey of reconnection and to pre-empt the need to process any challenging emotions that may arise along the way, it's essential we begin with some basic resourcing strategies.

One resource is an internal safe space – a place you can retreat to in your imagination as and when you choose, be it to seek refuge from stress or an over-active mind, or as a simple daily relaxation exercise.

Research consistently shows the power imagination plays in shaping the brain and body, as imagined events trigger biochemical, physiological and emotional responses that are identical to those that are real – it's more than daydreaming! This means that visualization, once disregarded as a pseudoscience, has now been shown to be a viable intervention for shaping our experience. In a University of Cincinnati study, a six-week follow-up showed chronic stroke patients who engaged in guided visualizations of moving the hand, arm and shoulder of their impaired side had significantly better functioning than the control group who did pure relaxation instead.[16] Even beyond aiding stroke recovery[17] and facilitating brain restoration,[18] intriguing findings arise. Volunteers who imagined flexing their finger multiple times daily exhibited a 35 per cent strength increase, compared to a 53 per cent increase through actual movement – that's just an 18 per cent difference between the two groups and yet it was through imagination alone![19] In a separate study, participants were divided into two groups: one physically played a piano sequence, whilst the other mentally rehearsed it. Remarkably, daily brain scans revealed changes to the finger muscle region in both groups, so much so that they were unable to distinguish the scans of those participants that had played the piano from those that had merely imagined playing.[20]

There is even research that has found the same network of brain activation in imagined exposure to threatening stimuli, such as that experienced in anxiety and PTSD, versus treatment via real extinction methods used in psychological therapy. This supports what psychologists have known for some time – that the imagination can be a great tool to eliminate fears and phobias, alter the way we respond to future situations and enhance decision-making and emotional regulation.[21]

Such findings challenge the boundary between imagination and reality and illustrate the power we have to consciously rewire our brain and transform our life experiences. For this reason, we'll be combining guided visualization with many of the exercises throughout this book, beginning right now, with setting up an inner sanctuary of safety for you and helping to connect you with a delightful sense of ease.

Visualizations use language that relates to imagery. Some people find it easy to visualize, but that's not true for everyone. So, if you're new to this work, struggle with visualization or are plagued by an overly analytical or cynical mind that brings in doubt, even if you see only darkness as you go through this exercise, continue to follow the directions and *imagine* you can see, as that way you're still sending out a powerful intention and will also benefit.

Safe Space Exercise

1. Find a comfortable space where you won't be disturbed. Close your eyes and place awareness into the body to connect with the breath.

2. Label any current thoughts, feelings or discomfort in the body, and imagine beaming them into a container of your choosing; be it a box, a cabinet or even a shipping container – whatever instinctively feels right. Close it or lock it up, and store away for later, so you can focus on the exercise.

3. Come back to the breath and bring to mind a time and place where you've felt safe and at peace (perhaps a special moment on a relaxing holiday). If you have nowhere specific, or have never felt safe, begin by imagining what elements might work and consciously construct your own peaceful scenario. (Exclude anyone you know from the scene as that can negatively impact the associations.)

4. Step into that place, seeing, hearing and feeling it as if you are there right now. Feel the sun on your skin, the wind in your hair – turn the dial up high on all your senses and notice the bodily sensations as you connect with the feelings.

5. Associate a word like peace, safety or freedom with this place so that, with repetition, that one word will be programmed to instantly take you straight back to that feeling.

Come back to the breath, open your eyes and bring those feelings with you into the next moments of your day. Return to this exercise as preparation for any potentially triggering exercises in the book, or use it to deactivate your stress-response system (more on this later) if you become emotionally activated. It can be particularly helpful if you feel overwhelmed by your emotions and need to refocus your attention elsewhere.

An extended version of this exercise is also available on my website (*page xxvi*), as well as in the audiobook.

Now you're resourced, let's take a moment to explore your current Self-connection. Because of our life experiences and conditioning, many of us tend to habitually over-identify with some levels of the Self and disengage from others – we may be 'overly emotional' or stuck in our logical thinking mind, for example. This focused attention in one direction limits how available we can be to the rest, creating disconnections elsewhere. This is particularly common if we have a history of trauma, as we're likely to subconsciously cut off from some elements of the Self as a protective mechanism.

If you're living in disconnect, you'll be likely to notice this playing out in many aspects of your life. Some areas will be working much better than others, and the quiz below will help bring to your awareness the specific levels of the Self that may need some additional attention.

Self-Connection Quiz

This true/false exercise has been developed through my clinical knowledge and client observations; it's not a scientifically validated research questionnaire. It's a valuable tool to help you 'zoom in' on aspects of Self-connection that we will work with in later exercises.

Instructions

Read through the following statements and answer whether you feel they're a true or false representation of where you find yourself in your life right *now*. Be sure to take care to highlight the correct column, as the true/false responses are intentionally not in the same position for every statement.

▲	I am often exhausted. I suffer from fatigue and a lack of energy, and find my sleep and health are suffering too.	True	False
★	I feel like my life has great meaning and purpose. I know what I want and why I'm here.	False	True
■	I constantly replay events and conversations in my mind, find it hard to switch off and struggle to sleep.	True	False
●	I isolate myself when times are tough (cancel plans, ignore calls/texts) – people don't know what's going on.	True	False
■	I really know my own mind, so I can make decisions easily and effortlessly.	False	True
●	I lose myself when around others – it's like I become more of them and less of me.	True	False
▲	I have a clean bill of health – no major health concerns for me.	False	True
■	I often struggle to remember things, especially details of my childhood.	True	False
★	I fully trust my instincts and act in accordance, knowing everything will work out.	False	True
♥	I am someone that's been plagued by anxiety and panic – life can be tough.	True	False
●	I acknowledge my own needs and ensure I have healthy boundaries with others.	False	True
♥	Sometimes my emotions can feel so overwhelming that I just don't know what to do.	True	False
▲	I take my body for granted and 'push on', overriding a need for rest. I always put everything else as a priority.	True	False
●	I trust others and turn to them in times of need.	False	True

★	I've never understood when people talk of healing and energetic connections – it's just not something I feel.	True	False
■	Sometimes it's like I'm living in a dream; I don't feel present and nothing feels real.	True	False
▲	I'm often out of touch with my body's signals: I forget to eat as I don't feel hungry/I don't feel full, so I overeat.	True	False
♥	I am present with my emotions, whatever they are, and then simply allow them to pass.	False	True
♥	I'm dissatisfied and despondent in life, yet lack any motivation to generate change.	True	False
★	I believe that I have all the resources I need within, so trust my inner guidance if needing answers/ making decisions.	False	True
▲	I'm plagued by aches and pains. I often feel 10 years older than I actually am.	True	False
●	I struggle to speak up and express my opinion. I don't really know what I stand for.	True	False
♥	It is easy for me to identify and understand how I am feeling in any given moment.	False	True
■	I find it hard to keep focus and concentration on tasks.	True	False
★	Sometimes I sense I should/shouldn't do certain things, but override my gut feeling and do them anyway.	True	False

Scoring

The table of statements has five different symbols on the left-hand side, representing the different levels of the Self introduced earlier. Look to the answers you gave and highlight *only* the responses that fall in the first column, then tally up the scores associated with each symbol and write them in the table on the next page.

Symbol	Level of Self	Score
▲	A disconnect/over-identification with the physical body	/5
♥	A disconnect/over-identification with the emotions	/5
■	A disconnect/over-identification with the thinking mind	/5
★	A disconnect/over-identification with intuition	/5
●	A disconnect/over-identification with relating to Self/Others	/5

How Did You Score?

You tend to score highest in the area (or areas) of Self you over-identify with or disconnect from – the level(s) at which your imbalance is expressed. Rank the categories from highest to lowest score and keep this in mind to help you focus on the areas needing more attention during the exercises to come.

Remember, though, that the levels are interrelated, so do keep in mind how each level may impact the rest. For example, my old Self would score five out of five on the physical body category. This is because I have habitually favoured my logical mind and switched off to what is occurring on the physical, emotional and spiritual levels. My body has therefore taken the brunt of the emotional turmoil I have suffered, which over time has come to mean numerous chronic and debilitating health conditions. This is the body having absorbed and suppressed all the split-off emotional energy generated by that thinking mind.

Let's take each level at a time and look at what your results could mean for you:

High Score with the Bodily Self

When overly identified with our thinking mind, we often become disconnected from what's happening within the body. This is also true when there is an imbalance at the emotional level, so the unexpressed vibrational energy associated with the emotions remains in the body. Over time, this suppression will take a toll and may find an outlet through mental or physical illnesses. If your score reveals a disconnect on the physical level of Self, it's likely you're out of tune with the body's innate signals, so are unlikely to attend to your physical needs or to notice when something isn't quite right.

It's likely that in your absence, the body is running on the hormones and biochemistry of survival, robbing you of any chance of producing what you need to remain healthy and well. So, whatever the reasoning behind not paying attention to your bodily Self, you're likely to be at/coming towards the stage when the body starts speaking more loudly through autoimmune conditions, allergic reactions, digestive complaints, chronic fatigue, dizziness, headaches, or maybe even more serious conditions such as cancer, diabetes or heart disease.

Alternatively, a high score in this category may show you're overly identified with what's happening in the body and may feel it is 'letting you down' as your energy is sapped, you suffer from fatigue, joint and muscle pain, and most likely struggle with your sleep.

High Score with the Emotional Self

There's likely to be limited joy and peace in your life when you have an imbalance in your emotional world, as you're either totally numb or only able to access those heavy, lower-vibrational frequencies that manifest in depression, grief, anxiety, fear, panic, stress and anger.

These frequencies also relate to your thoughts, which, as life might feel out of your control, are likely to perpetuate how you feel.

Life is a struggle when there is discord on the emotional level of Self. It can be hard to be present with your emotions, as you're likely to feel overwhelmed by stress, anxiety and panic – the world does not feel safe with an over-identification with lower-vibrational emotions.

If you're split off from this element of the Self, it can be hard to identify with how you *are* feeling, as when you cut off from one feeling, you tend to cut off from them all. This doesn't mean they don't exist, however, and the energy build-up in the body can not only manifest as illness, but also, due to the subconscious effort used to keep the emotional floodgates firmly closed, to limited life-force being available to engage fully with life, leading to a general despondency and disconnection from others.

High Score with the Thinking Self

If you scored highly in this category, then you tend to be preoccupied by your thoughts, replaying past hurts, hypervigilant to what might go wrong in the present and burdened by future fears. You may have developed some symptoms of a mental health condition, or even have a diagnosis. You tend to rely heavily on logic to make decisions, and as it can be hard to switch off from your thoughts, your sleep can often be negatively impacted, making any catastrophic thinking far worse.

If, on the other hand, you have *disconnected* from your thinking mind, you may struggle to really know and express your own thoughts and opinions. As a result, you can be easily influenced by others and struggle to make decisions. It can be hard to stay focused and concentrate on conversations or on tasks you're meant to be doing. This is because you have limited presence of mind, which can lead to trouble with memory recall as well.

High Score with the Intuitive-Self

If you're disconnected from this aspect of the Self, it can be hard to trust in your own 'gut' for decision-making, so you get stuck in analysis paralysis or seek guidance from elsewhere. You may find this undermines your self-confidence, self-belief and sense of autonomy over your life, as you become dependent on others for direction and lose sight of the fact that you have the capability to facilitate change. With a life limited to the logical, it can be hard to see past the concrete and generate opportunities beyond that which is constructed by the mind. This lack of connection with the creative flow of infinite possibility robs you of a sense of purpose and meaning, so life loses a dimension of wonder.

If this is instead a level of Self you currently over-identify with, it's likely you too outsource your decision-making, but this time to an invisible realm. With less grounding in physical reality, you can lose touch with what it means to have a human experience and begin neglecting the needs of your physical body and mind, having handed over your destiny to a higher power or predestined fate.

High Score Relating to Self/Others

Not only does an imbalance within the Self-system result in a disconnection from fundamentally important parts that make up who we are and how we function in the world, but it can also limit our ability to connect with other people on a relational level. We can only be as present with another person to the degree that we can be present with ourselves.

If you have scored highly in this category, you're likely to be disconnected from or preoccupied with your Self, which in turn impacts your ability to be present in relation to others. You can often feel less engaged with those around you, leading to an externalized sense of separation that mirrors that of your internal state.

It can be hard to know who you are, what you stand for or how to address your own needs, as you tend to lose yourself as your energy and awareness goes out to others. It becomes hard to know what's theirs and what's yours. With a lack of boundaries and a poor sense of Self, it's easy to over-identify with the thoughts, feelings, needs and desires of another person.

As well as being absent from the Self when present with others, it can also be the case that when too present with the Self, or overly identified with it, you have limited resources available to be present with another. You may find that others disconnect from you as they sense this lack of depth within the relationship. Being more focused on yourself when relating to others can feel safe, but can also make it hard to trust others in times of need, so you avoid contact when you perhaps need it most. You can remain isolated and alone as a result.

So, when there is an imbalance on this level of the Self, you can be present with others but absent from your Self, or vice versa. Either way, your relationships become unsatisfactory, leaving you feeling separate and alone, or perhaps misunderstood and not seen for who you truly are.

Reflecting on Your Self-Connection Quiz Score

I wonder what insights you've gained from engaging with this quiz. Take a moment to think through where you feel you might have been over- and under-identifying with those different levels of the Self.

Begin by writing down in your journal why that imbalance might be there. Have you shut off from your emotions because you grew up hearing that 'Big girls don't cry'? Or were you constantly praised for being 'so clever and bright' and so learnt to focus on your mind to the detriment of all else? Maybe it was the body that became your focus, as you were only really noticed when you became ill. Take a moment to think of the different narratives you've experienced and the impact they've had in denying you access to a fully integrated Self.

Now take note of how that has limited your life. What have you missed out on as a result, and how does all this impact how you relate with yourself and others?

Once you have gained this awareness, look to what you can start to release now. What key areas need to be brought into conscious awareness, and what do you need to focus on to gain more balance and harmony, both within and between these different levels of the Self? Where do you need to breathe in more life, and what do you need to release and realign? We will look at this more deeply in Part II, but for now, welcome in your own realizations.

//

Becoming aware of your current truth and the beliefs, opinions and experiences you carry is of great importance, as it will impact what reality you're able to see, and thus what outcomes are readily available to you. Ultimately, whether you're able to embrace and meet your whole authentic Self as a multi-dimensional being – body, heart, mind and soul.

With this in mind, I invite you to consider how open you are to experiences beyond the bounds of belief. There is much, *much* more out there for us to learn than can be found in a textbook or at a school or university. It's through drawing upon your *inner*-tuition (the guidance that speaks from within) that a limitless journey of self-discovery and self-healing can begin.

A full exploration of psychic phenomena and 'otherworldly' teachings are beyond the intention and scope of this book, but we will be drawing on my experience of these phenomena along the way.

We will take this journey one stage at a time:

1. First you will be eating up all the knowledge and wisdom necessary for growth.

2. Then, having created the conditions for your cocoon of change, you'll be fully integrating and grounding each aspect of your past-, present- and future-Self possibilities.

3. Finally, you'll emerge into a new, fully connected life, one that encompasses all the necessary tools and wisdom for physical, emotional, mental, spiritual and relational wellbeing.

Seriously, what other choice can you make?

Let's reflect...

Your Current Timeline – Remaining as You Are

If you were to place this book back on the shelf right now and decide to remain as your present-Self, the one unconsciously conditioned to repeat the problems of the past, what is the future that lies in wait?

Ask yourself:

▲ What does this future look like?

▲ Is this how I want my life to unfold?

▲ Would I *choose* to spend my time this way?

▲ Is this how I want my life to *feel*?

Take a moment to ponder the above questions in your journal. Is this *really* the future-Self you wish to become? Then, ask yourself:

▲ If not, why not? What's getting in the way?

▲ What would it take to let go of the past and embrace a new timeline that connects with a future-Self of your choosing?

▲ What might you need to release that is standing in the way of aligning your energy, thoughts and actions with this?

▲ Who do you need to let go of to become that new identity – for example, do you currently identify as an ill person, a lazy one, a failure?

▲ Could that person have the life you're wishing to create, or do you need to become someone new?

▲ What do you need in practical terms to help achieve it?

▲ Imagine waiting at the pearly gates, reviewing your life and the decisions you've made. If you were there now, would you be at peace or ravaged by regret? If regret, then check if you've been consciously constructing your life.

This book gives you the opportunity to release yourself from a future moulded by the past and to consciously generate something better. To do so, you'll need an outcome in mind encompassing all the levels of the Self, otherwise how will you know when you get there?

Your New Timeline – Setting Your Destination Co-ordinates

Perhaps you don't yet know which direction you'd like your life to take. If so, don't worry, by the end of this book you certainly will. That's why we're dropping it into your awareness now – to generate the breadcrumbs that will take you there. Your destination may evolve as you gain new insight and knowledge from the book. That's part of the process. In fact, I invite you to occasionally check in with your desired future to ensure you're still on track and to amend the route if necessary. In doing so, you're building powerful networks in your brain and setting the very clear energetic intention that this is where you're heading.

For now, explore where you'd like life to take you, then brainstorm what might need to happen for you to get there. Just like with the satnav in your car, reaching your desired outcome hinges on the co-ordinates given, so if there's no accurate destination or route, you can't exactly complain if life leads you to a dead-end!

Reflect on:

▲ **Aspirations**: How do you wish to transform your life? In what areas/direction would you prefer your life to go? What will you think/feel/experience in relation to this?

▲ **Purpose**: Know your 'why'. What is the purpose behind this change? What does it mean to you to get there? What impact will it have beyond you?

▲ **Identity**: Who do you need to be to become this person - what needs to change? What aspects of your current Self do you need to harness/let go of/adapt/develop?

▲ **Values and beliefs**: What values and beliefs will you need to hold about yourself, others, and the world to align with the life you envision and to guide your decisions/actions?

▲ **Skills and knowledge**: In what areas do you need to develop and grow, and what new expertise, knowledge, and skills are necessary for these future endeavours?

▲ **Relationships**: What existing supportive relationships can you nurture and where can you seek new connections that align with your new values and aspirations?

▲ **Environment**: What physical and social environments will contribute positively to your wellbeing and new desired lifestyle and identity? What needs to change?

This isn't about denying or disowning who you are now, it's about taking back the reins and consciously directing your life in accordance with the future of your choosing.

This is exactly what I did when deciding I would win the publishing contract on offer at the Hay House Writer's Workshop. My destination was holding my book at a Hay House event, having previously won the contract. Notice I selected an event *after* the competition, because for that chosen event to happen, I'd already have won! Consciously re-experiencing this on all the levels of the Self, I acted, thought, felt and resonated exactly as if it had already happened. I even researched the telephone area code for Michelle Pilley, Managing Director of Hay House UK, so I could be sure to answer her call making the announcement, which, by the way, came the very moment I pulled into a restaurant car park for a meal I'd pre-booked to celebrate the win with my two daughters.

Now, I'm aware this confidence could sound a little conceited, but this wasn't about me, it was about my life purpose, which is *to help people to help themselves*. Don't get me wrong – you can't just conjure up something and expect it will materialize. It has to match your energetic frequency and life path, plus you need to put in the work. I researched, read and wrote day and night to complete that proposal – I gave it my all! Had I not done so, I wouldn't have won, had I not finished on time, I wouldn't have won, and had I not attended the workshop, again, I wouldn't have won. I 'became an author' mentally, physically, emotionally and spiritually, knowing my new identity had to start in the *now* for me to be a match with my future-Self as an author.

The point is, if I can do this, then so can you!

So, let's get specific:

Planning Your Desired Outcome

Choose a desired outcome for your future-Self.

Start with the end result and work your way back, noting the steps you have taken to get there.

Break down the route into manageable parts and map out what's needed for you to find your way into that future. How will you get there? When? What help or preparation will you need, if any? How will you get that?

Generate a plan of action. What do you need to do, be, believe, feel?

Put this plan on paper in words or images. You could even record yourself saying it on your phone. However you do it:

▲   Make it as detailed as possible.

▲   Word it in the positive – rather than 'I don't want this terrible fatigue and pain', write: 'I am full of vitality and health.' Connect with what you *actually* want.

▲   Write in the present tense – for example, 'I am', rather than 'I want'. The latter is a frequency of striving rather than one of certainty.

Language is only one aspect of the frequency or energy you're generating; your thoughts, emotions and actions also play a significant role in shaping your overall vibration and in attracting what you want to call into your life.

Well done! You've just locked in some reference points to find along your journey and primed the body, mind and heart for what's to come next. Now, when the time for change comes, it will feel more familiar and safe, especially if you've already been replaying it. We'll revisit this exercise at the end of the book to complete the process of re-programming your timeline, so you'll need to keep this future outcome alive until then. Really *feeling* the positive emotions of this future-Self helps to draw it to you like a magnet.

Meanwhile, we must gather the knowledge and theory that can make this future manifest and release the blocks and conditioning from the past that can prevent your progression.

But first we need to take a closer look at where so many of us are right now.

CHAPTER 2

AN ABSENCE OF SELF – MIND, BODY AND SOUL(LESS) LIVING

Abandonment of the Self has its roots firmly planted in the unspoken constructs of the Western society and culture we live in today, as we strive to fit in, to feel loved and to be accepted. Materialism is rewarded and self-gain is prioritized over optimum health and happiness, as we seek to consume for comfort, to silence all suffering and to medicate the mundane.

With our current technological advances, never before have we had such an amazing opportunity for connectedness, the vast majority of us spending hours each day plugged into the internet. Tempted and tantalized by constant engagement, we have the entire world at our fingertips 24 hours a day, seven days a week. Yet this is nothing more than a cruel deception, a misleading façade we need to shatter to free ourselves from purely living in the mind instead of exploring reality as a multi-dimensional being – body, heart, mind *and* soul. Rather than bringing us closer and providing connection, all this noise in our external world merely serves to silence the whispers from our inner landscape. Whilst we can often pay attention to how connected we feel to others, staying in touch with friends, with family, with co-workers, rarely do we make the space or time to connect with ourselves – our habitual thoughts, our emotions, our bodily sensations, inner knowing, likes and dislikes. So, we lose touch with our true essence.

Why do we live this way? We disconnect from our true Self (and others) when it becomes too painful to be who we are, when it becomes too painful to live our lives and when our life path reveals that which is too painful to see.

This denial of who we truly are and how we truly feel also brings forth an external persona we typically refer to as 'the ego' or 'the false Self'. This is the Self we present to the world. Many of us actually begin to think this counterfeit caricature is who we are. We're so caught up in the façade that we fail to notice that our entire existence is built upon false foundations. For many, this is only ever revealed once the walls come tumbling down, be it through chronic mental or physical illness, relationship discord or an unexplained sense of dissatisfaction and disillusionment. As our authenticity crumbles, each time we suppress our inner truth, each time we give away our power, silence our voice or trade our integrity to remain in favour, another part of the Self dies within.

It's my belief that one of the fundamental reasons for the current wellness deficit in our modern world is this disconnection from the Self, specifically a disconnection from the spiritual and an over-identification with the mental, emotional and physical. Moreover, our fast-paced, technologically advanced culture exposes us to an internal and external environment full of toxic energies and vibrations that can wreak havoc on us physically, mentally, emotionally and spiritually.

Look around you. Can you see how unhappy and unfulfilled we are as a society? It's no secret that as a collective, we have never been more alone and more mentally and physically ill, because instead of listening to the wisdom of our body as it communicates its dis-ease and dis-trust to us, we seek to silence it through strategies such as denial, suppression and distraction. In doing so, we're inadvertently priming it to speak ever louder, until we have no choice but to listen – and when our body speaks our truth, it speaks in a language of pain, panic disorder, cardiovascular disease, respiratory illness, diabetes and cancer, to name a few.

In 2021, the World Health Organization (WHO) reported that non-communicable diseases, such as cardiovascular disease, cancer, diabetes and chronic respiratory diseases, were responsible for 71 per cent of all global deaths, with 41 million people dying each year as a result.[1] These diseases also account for the premature death of over 80 per cent of people aged between 30 and 69 years old. This document also highlighted that depression affects 264 million people globally,[2] with treatment and support services inaccessible to many. Sadly, it's no surprise, therefore, that an estimated 700,000 people die by suicide each year,[3] and for every successful suicide, there are approximately 20 attempts that fail.[4]

Fortunately, we have much more power over our ability to heal than the current medical model would have us believe.

THE MIND–BODY CONNECTION

In recent years, we've accumulated more and more research supporting the connection between the mind and body, despite Western medicine, in theory and practice, treating them as separate entities. This is an all-important finding, showing not only how our mind can influence our physiology but also how our physiology can influence our mind. This provides an encouraging foundation for the premise that we have within us the power to alter our health and wellbeing – both to our detriment and for our gain.

Studies in the areas of psycho-neuro-immunology and psycho-neuro-endocrinology have provided evidence of links between the immune system and the brain, and have also shown that, crucially, our emotions affect our levels of immunity.[5] You only need to look at the recent global Covid-19 health crisis to see the importance of such findings, which point to the necessity to connect with factors within our own control that can impact the prevention of and recovery from illness and disease. Strangely enough, the notion that the brain and body are interconnected and our psychological and emotional wellbeing could have an effect on our physical health had been totally dismissed for many years prior to this. That was until clinical studies such as those conducted by Dr Candace Pert,[6] and Professor George Soloman[7] gave more support to the notion that our emotions are linked with our immune system and therefore have a significant influence on the progression of disease.

Such research helps us to acknowledge the link between our mind, emotions and physical body and recognize that the immune system, endocrine system, nervous system and brain all interact. This helps us move beyond the notion of illness and disease having a purely physical root and towards a holistic approach and the promotion of self-healing.

This evidence of a body–mind connection also bolsters the claim of this book: that through embracing this connection with an awareness on all the levels of the Self and across the timeline that spans our past, present and future, we have the power to help and heal ourselves, enabling us to evolve as individuals and as a society, rather than remaining in a perpetual state of avoidance, apathy and disconnect.

You see, whilst Western scientific and medical systems often prioritize a disease model of health and fail to promote self-healing, in some respects this has also been true of psychology. Some psychologists, though not all, may now link the impact of our thoughts, feelings and behaviours to physical maladies; however, what is less common are the psychologists who take this one step further and bring a body–mind–heart–*soul* approach to their life and work.

I'm suggesting that we can expand our views and treatments by bringing *all* the elements together. We don't need to exclude conventional medicine or choose spirituality over science, we need to marry the two together, with an open regard for that which isn't yet measurable.

For an example of this, we need only look at the way mindfulness, a tool originating in Buddhist spiritual teachings, has gone from being frowned upon as unscientific to, following numerous research studies, being hailed as a beneficial intervention for a wide range of health concerns. In particular, a 2013 meta-analysis reviewing 200 studies that involved more than 12,000 participants showed this to be true for anxiety, depression, pain and chronic illness, to name but a few.[8]

We even have research that attests to the benefits of spiritual practice. In studies comparing participants with a 'high' versus 'low' spiritual practice, MRI imaging has revealed a more spiritually awakened brain to be healthier and have thicker and stronger pathways in the very regions that weaken and wither in the brains of those who are depressed.[9] Now, based on the statistics for depression and suicide given at the beginning of this chapter, this is clearly an important finding to consider further.

THE PHYSICAL SELF

Before we delve further into the deeply spiritual aspects of the amazing journey that awaits you, we must look at the physical Self. After all, many of you are likely to have been drawn to this book because you're struggling physically, perhaps with headaches, body aches, digestive issues or mysterious physical symptoms that medical doctors simply cannot correctly diagnose or treat. While you may be able to make a loose connection between your life choices and some of your symptoms – too much spicy food leads to indigestion, a lack of sleep contributes to headaches, and perhaps you've 'inherited' your body pains from your mum – the underlying reason for these symptoms may be much tougher to pin down, and may be rooted in trauma.

Stress and Trauma

Stress and trauma are often seen as separate issues in our culture. Often 'stress' is used to describe our reaction to everyday annoyances, pressures and anxieties, from crying babies to looming deadlines. For some, it's even something to brag about – a sign of how busy or important they are. 'Trauma', on the other hand, is often reserved for catastrophic events or traumatic experiences that haunt us and leave a long-term psychological scar.

I know what you're thinking. You're thinking, *Hold on a minute – I haven't experienced trauma. I'm just stressed out, burnt-out, needing a break.* But what would you say if I told you that being constantly overworked and sleep-deprived could have the same effect on your mind and body as post-traumatic stress disorder (PTSD)? Just because you might not have experienced a major trauma such as a war or famine, a natural disaster or abuse, you're still affected by the events that have happened to you, and even those you've witnessed over the course of your life. Not only that, but research shows you may even inherit trauma – it can be passed down genetically, behaviourally and energetically (*see Chapter 8*). Even the culture into which you're born imprints its wounds into your energetic blueprint, both before and after your birth. So you may not have lived through a major traumatic experience yourself, but the body may be responding as though you have. Trauma is something we must all have an awareness of if we're to release ourselves from its subconscious hold.

As trauma can be a universal experience from the collective, inherited through our parents or our culture as well as encountered at an individual level, it's clear that there is likely to be some unresolved trauma permeating the levels of your being, and the impact on the body is always the same – an activation of the stress-response system.

Both stress and trauma activate this system, and they can have equally severe effects on our mental and physical health. That's right, your mind and body don't differentiate between stress and trauma. So that angry email from your boss will activate the survival response you'll rely on if you're ever caught up in the middle of a bank raid at gunpoint.

More on the stress-response system later, but a stress response is essentially a neurological, physiological and psychological response triggered by a *perceived* threat. That perception will vary from person to person. Elizabeth Stanley, PhD, in her book *Widen the Window*,[10] talks of our individual ability to handle stress as a window, with the amount of stress we can tolerate being directly proportionate to the size of the window. The size of our window is determined by such factors as our capacity to cope, find solutions and regulate our emotions. The window narrows with exposure to chronic stress and trauma.

I personally use the analogy of a bucket filling up. We travel through our lives with our own individual bucket holding our thoughts, emotions and stress. The capacity of our bucket will initially be set at birth, influenced by factors such as the genetic material passed down by our parents. So, if there's already trauma in our ancestry, at birth our bucket may already be half full. Any difficult childhood experiences with caregivers that negatively influence our bond or dysregulate our stress hormonal system will take up more of the bucket, as will each and every unprocessed traumatic or stressful life event from that point onwards – until it overflows!

The Survival Brain

What is happening in our brain when we are stressed?

The workings of the brain are often explained by the Triune Brain Theory proposed by neuroscientist Paul MacLean in the 1960s.[11] It suggests that the human brain is made up of three evolutionarily distinct parts, each with its own set of functions and characteristics:

1. The surface (neocortex), known as 'the thinking brain', enables higher cognitive functions such as sensory perception, language, reasoning and planning. These activities are mostly conscious and voluntary and associated with primates.

2. Below the surface lies 'the emotional brain', also known as the mammalian brain or limbic system. This area is thought to be responsible for behavioural and emotional responses, along with memory processing, as it consists of the hypothalamus and the hippocampus.

3. Finally, there is 'the survival brain', which consists of the brainstem and the cerebellum. This is the more primitive part of the brain, responsible for regulating our basic survival functions, such as breathing, heart rate and hunger, most of which are not under our conscious control, along with instinctual behaviours, balance and movement.

While this theory has been influential in both neuroscience and popular culture, it's important to note that it's now considered by many researchers to be oversimplified. More recent research has shown that the brain is much more adaptive than this and uses processes that involve multiple parts working together in complex ways.[12] Instead of three relatively independent brain regions, there are interconnected networks said to control various aspects of our thoughts, emotions and bodily functions. These networks can adapt and change over time to help us predict and respond to changing circumstances in our environment. By working together, they help our brain maintain a stable internal state, regulate our emotions and support our ability to think, learn and make decisions.

The Stress-Response System

So, instead of referring to 'the survival brain' when talking of stress, trauma and the fight-or-flight response, based on a new adaptive brain model, I will use the term 'stress-response system'.

At a subconscious level, the nervous system is automatically evaluating safety and risk in the environment in a process called neuroception, a term introduced by neurologist and psychologist Dr Stephen Porges when he presented Polyvagal Theory,[13] a framework that builds on our understanding of the autonomic nervous system (ANS) with the addition of the social engagement system[14] (we will touch on this shortly).

Neuroception is the brain and body's way of detecting whether a person or a situation is safe. When a danger is perceived, the stress-response system, designed to help us respond to short-term threats and recover afterwards, engages our autonomic nervous system, which controls our heart rate, breathing, hormones and digestion, and prepares us for action.

The ANS has two branches: the sympathetic nervous system (SNS), which is responsible for turning stress activation on, and the parasympathetic nervous system (PSNS), which is responsible for turning it off. Dr Porges has more recently added a third system, social engagement, which refers to the ability to connect with others and regulate emotions and behaviour in social situations.

Sympathetic Nervous System:

- Associated with the fight-or-flight response

- Activated in response to perceived danger or threat

- Triggers a release of adrenaline and other stress hormones, leading to increased heart rate, blood pressure and respiratory rate, as well as other physiological changes that prepare the body to respond to the threat

Parasympathetic Nervous System:

- Associated with the 'rest and digest' response

- Activated when the body perceives that it is safe and can conserve energy

- Helps to slow down heart rate, breathing and other physiological processes, promoting relaxation, recovery and restoration

Social Engagement System:

- Associated with the ability to connect and co-regulate emotions and behaviours with others in a safe and social context

- Activated in response to perceived social safety, i.e. when a person feels secure, welcome and not under threat in relation to others

- Promotes physiological responses aimed at facilitating effective social interactions, engagement and bonding through relaxed facial expressions, appropriate vocal tones and gestures that enhance communication and empathy

Designed to mobilize a lot of energy at once, our stress-response system reacts to perceived danger by speeding up our heart rate, slowing down digestion and increasing oxygen flow to our brain. After such heavy activation, body and brain then need to recover, so our brain, hormones, immune system and nervous system can return to a healthy baseline. This recovery is managed by a process called allostasis. However, in the same way that you can't control your instinctive stress response, you can't control recovery. For it to happen, your nervous system needs to perceive safety.

Chronic stress and unresolved trauma can impede this recovery, because they simply don't allow us to feel safe. Under these conditions, our stress-response system is always activated, so an allostatic load builds up that can't be discharged, resulting in our body permanently focusing on short-term survival instead of long-term health, producing short-acting stress hormones such as cortisol and adrenaline and slowing down the production of long-acting growth, repair and reproductive hormones.

When the stress-response system remains activated like this, we'll have trouble recovering after trauma and stressful life events. Important functions of our nervous, hormone and immune systems become impaired, and so our body, heart and brain become dysregulated, priming us for mental and physical illness and disease. This happens often in our modern culture, when we're constantly under pressure, have high anxiety or are sleep-deprived, for example. In all these cases, our environment, internal and external, is actively preventing our mind and body from coming to rest. Safety isn't found and so the rest and repair mode of the PSNS cannot be activated, and our social engagement system also remains offline.

Addressing how well your autonomic nervous system is regulating your physiological and emotional response to stress and danger is of paramount importance if you intend to become the future-Self you have envisaged. Any attempt to change when under the influence of stress and trauma can only be viewed through a lens tinted by threat, so instead of enjoying the triumph of transformation, you'll remain disconnected and living life on high alert!

It's also important to note that the stress-response system doesn't distinguish between real and imagined threats,[15] so any ongoing negative thoughts, whether based on reality or imagined, can be just as dysregulating and damaging to the mind and body as a traumatic life event itself. Just think about that for a moment!

Trauma

Dr Dan Siegal, a clinical professor of psychiatry at the UCLA School of Medicine, defines trauma in the simplest of ways: 'an experience we have that overwhelms our capacity to cope'. I like this definition, as trauma and stress take many forms, and we're each impacted by an experience relative to the meaning we place upon it and the degree to which we feel helpless or overwhelmed. So, trauma may take the form of neglect, be it physical abandonment, emotional abuse or a general air of disinterest. It can include chronic illness, the death of a loved one, ridicule by a caregiver during childhood, even the loss of a promotion, witnessing harm to another, a lost friendship or inescapable harassment at school or work. It's all shaped by our individual life circumstances, the capacity of our bucket and our perception of the event.

Whatever form it takes, trauma impacts every layer of our being, including the energetic level, as our vibrational frequency meets interference from the energetic impact of a stronger, denser energy field. That's why we can often feel like we've been *hit by a bus* when sudden trauma is upon us, and why corresponding aches and pains may follow.

Trauma affects the body in a myriad of complex ways, but most difficulties seem to come back to the activation of the stress-response system. When the stress response is activated, research indicates that we're more likely to develop a whole host of physical and psychological conditions – depression, anxiety, obsessive-compulsive disorder (OCD), post-traumatic stress disorder (PTSD), insomnia, heart attack, cancer, obesity and stroke, to name but a few.

Chronic stress and trauma can lead to two types of response in the body: an over-active response (hyper-arousal) and an under-active response (hypo-arousal). Someone with an over-active response is easily activated. Their reactions to life events may seem outsized to those who haven't experienced direct trauma. You know when you're in a hyper-aroused state, as you'll tend to display certain characteristics that involve an excess of energy, you'll have intense emotional reactions, might have a sense of wanting to run away and may be more prone to emotional outbursts, defensiveness and anger. If defaulting to this over-active response, you may also be more likely to experience anxiety, addictions, impulsivity, hypervigilance or obsessive-compulsive thoughts or behaviours.

Hypo-arousal can occur following an extended period of hyper-arousal, when our adrenaline and cortisol have been activated for so long that we just crash into a dissociative or shutdown state. Someone with an under-active response may disengage emotionally from themselves and others and walk around feeling disconnected and numb. You'll know if you're experiencing a hypo-aroused response, as you're likely to feel exhausted and depressed, to struggle with your memory and cognitive processes, and often just want to shut out the world and sleep all the time. You're often not consciously present to the experience of your everyday life, as you're sapped of all life energy and only just manage to function by running on autopilot.

Sometimes the emotional charge of a traumatic memory will show up in the body as dysfunction, pressure or pain. When suppressed, the associated emotional energy gets trapped in the body, and not only lives on in the physical and cognitive patterns that result but can often generate mental or physical illness or disease until the connected trauma is released. I see this so often in my clinic, and sadly, my experience shows how predictable this can be. If we don't express the emotional charge and complete the trauma response, then the body will speak our truth until we listen.

So, whilst we may have been taught that many of our illnesses have been inherited, our genes do not solely determine our destiny. The disconnect within the body-heart-mind-soul is a much larger contributor to stress, burnout and disease than we may realize. As a matter of fact, for those of you who haven't yet come into an awareness of how the lived experience of your past deeply affects your present, stress and burnout may actually be the *surface* symptoms – the first clues to this underlying issue.

Can you spot yourself in the descriptions above? No matter which type of response the body has, the important thing to note is that it is having a response. The body is communicating that there is some underlying trauma, disconnection or need that must be dealt with. The body is speaking to you.

Are you ready to listen?

THE BODY SCAN

Now we're going to connect you with your physical body. In the preceding chapter we discussed how important it is to be connected at all the levels of the Self, and that connectedness begins with the physical body. It's through this sensing vessel that we feel our emotions and can ground ourselves in order to connect to the higher energetic realms, so choosing to consciously become mindful of the body is fundamental to your ability to heal on many levels.

This practice of conducting a mindful body scan will not only help you to gain more body awareness. Amongst many other positive benefits, body scans alone have been found to significantly increase wellbeing,[16] decrease anxiety, depression and stress,[17] improve sleep[18] and significantly increase parasympathetic activity.[19] So this simple practice, when done regularly, can help to switch off the stress-response system and mitigate the health implications that could result.

Now this practice does have the potential to become triggering for people who have experienced trauma, have anxieties relating to the body or who experience pain, so do give yourself some self-compassion and care. You may wish to complete the safe space exercise (*page 16*) beforehand, or even seek help and guidance from a professional if you feel you might need additional support.

The body scan is effectively a mindfulness practice that involves bringing attention to different parts of the body to observe any sensations or feelings that arise, without judgement. The goal isn't to change the body's state or induce relaxation, but to simply be present with whatever arises in the moment, and then move onto the next body part. I have adapted this exercise to incorporate an awareness of the energetic body also.

So, let's begin:

The Body Scan

Find a quiet and comfortable place to sit or lie down where you won't be disturbed for around 10-15 minutes.

Close your eyes or soften your gaze, whilst dropping your awareness into the body and onto your breath.

Take a few slow, deep breaths, allowing your mind to settle. During the practice your mind will wander. That's perfectly natural – just gently escort it back to the anchor of the breath and the sensations present in the body.

Begin the scan by directing your attention to the soles of your feet, feeling the contact with the floor, and simply observe the sensations.

Pause…

Now, as you continue to focus your awareness on your feet and the breath moving in and out of the body, imagine the breath moving in and out through the bottom of your feet.

Pause…

Take your time and pay attention to any sensations, without judging them or trying to change them. Just be there and remain present with a conscious awareness of the feet.

Repeat this process for other areas of the body, gradually working your way up through the legs, the front and back of the torso, the chest, the arms, face, the head, whilst simply remaining aware to what's present in each moment.

When you've worked your way through the *whole* body, extend your awareness out into the space around the body. What do you notice in the energy surrounding the physical body? Explore the sensations here also.

Finally, when you're ready, bring your attention back to the breath. Take a few gentle deep breaths, slowly open your eyes and journal on your experience.

CHAPTER 3

THE COST OF
A DISCONNECTED SELF

I know this cost only too well.

It took repeatedly clawing my way back to survival after losing my health to one debilitating illness after another.

It took the trauma of becoming the only surviving member of my immediate family as death wiped out each generation one by one.

It took letting go of the 20-year relationship with my husband in favour of becoming a single mum, whilst running two businesses and literally building the house we were yet to call a home.

It took all of that and much, much more for me to *finally* wake up to the realization that each and every time I found myself in a place of pain and suffering, each and every time the spark to my fire was extinguished, and each and every time I had nothing left to give, it was *always* preceded by a substantial disconnection from the Self.

I remember when I first became aware of this disconnect. I'd been working in a leadership development role in corporate HR at Reuters Ltd since leaving university. There I was, commuting on the zombie express into London day after day. Neatly pressed trouser suits from Joseph, bag and shoes from Russell and Bromley – I made sure I looked the part. To the outside world, it was clear I had a great career ahead of me. Yet behind that crisp façade, all I felt was pain. I was burnt-out, bereft of all life-force, desperately pushing through each and every day, hanging on as if my very existence was dependent upon it. The threat of tarnishing my image of corporate perfection hung over me, so there was no time or space to acknowledge the illness that was taking hold, but most damningly, there was no compassion or love from the unrelenting tyrant that dominated my world – my mind. I just had to keep pushing through, but to do that I had to disconnect further from my reality – I had to disconnect further from the Self.

I'd already spent years challenging and erasing my lifelong esoteric encounters, turning instead to the shelter of scientific explanation. I was ashamed and embarrassed to own and express this more intuitive aspect of my Self; instead, I suppressed my truth and placated the eye-rollers, the sceptics and the outright disbelievers by denying the very aspects of my Self that made me uniquely me.

This disregard of my physical, emotional, mental and spiritual needs in pursuit of conforming to externally defined notions of success brought with it profound consequences that at the time I just wasn't prepared to see.

We all do this: we form an idea of who we should and shouldn't be based on the beliefs, opinions, external conditioning and cultural, social and media constructs we've been exposed to and internalized along the way. We then split off those parts of ourselves that we believe may act as a magnet for negative judgement, and dim our light rather than shine as who we are. Through this pruning of the Self, we gradually mould ourselves and our lives into a shape that no longer fits. We no longer resemble who we truly are and lose sight of all we could have become had we allowed in a little Self-acceptance.

Dimming those aspects of the Self and trying to crawl back into our cocoon comes at a cost. For me, that initially came in the form of my first pituitary tumour, diagnosed at the age of 22. I wonder what that cost has been for *you*. I wonder where that gentle pruning began and where you're now playing life small as a result. To what lengths have *you* gone to remain safe in your self-imposed cage rather than embracing a life full of freedom?

Do you ever feel that you're beset by challenge after challenge and unable to enjoy even the simplest of things life has to offer? Or, instead of basking in the sunshine of self-satisfaction at having achieved a personal goal, you somehow find yourself devoured by a darkness that emerges from the depths of self-desertion?

Be it physical illness, mental malaise or emotional exhaustion, when not living in alignment with your truth, when disconnected from the reality of who you truly are and when functioning on an autopilot that's rooted in your past conditioning, all too often the outcome is physical, emotional, mental, spiritual and even relational disorders, disconnection and disharmony, leaving you destined to live a lacklustre life.

As well as a hyper prolactinoma, a benign tumour of the pituitary gland that was secreting the hormone prolactin, I simultaneously received the diagnoses of reactive hypoglycaemia and endometriosis and was treated with medication that caused such serious side-effects and corresponding complications that I eventually stopped taking it entirely. What was actually needed was a time for self-reflection, where I could develop the awareness required for a conscious reconnection with all the levels of my existence – a necessary process that would enable me to fully heal and to recover.

You could assume that after facing all my challenges, I would naturally act in accordance with the profound insight that they brought forward and choose not to abandon the Self again. Sadly not! I knew what was happening and what I needed to do, but it took repeated lessons over many more years for me to take ownership of my part in creating my life's difficulties and to act without disconnecting from the Self once again! There's a big difference between *knowing* something intellectually and actually *doing it* for yourself!

Sadly, I see this all too often in my office. I can always tell when clients have stopped 'doing the work' – first the meditation goes, then the hours at work creep up, there's no time for movement and the healthy eating drops off. Before you know it, they're back feeling anxious, depressed or burnt-out, and failing to notice it's because they've stopped making the lifestyle choices that contributed towards keeping them well.

In our fast-paced society, it's all too easy to sacrifice the Self once a crisis is over and switch to a disconnected approach to life – one where the focus is 'out there' on anyone or anything that shouts a little bit louder than our own Self. But again, this comes at a cost. We slip back onto autopilot and begin setting ourselves up for the next difficult encounters – the next reminders to take the lessons on board and truly learn.

It was only through finally recognizing the necessity to support Self-awareness, cease Self-abandonment and surrender to Self-acceptance that I was able to overcome my difficulties and find freedom in life's flow.

Only through embracing my authentic Self at every level of my being and fully acknowledging and releasing the many years of pain and suffering my past-Self had endured was I able to see the irrefutable truth: that for me, the most detrimental death of all was not the loss of those I loved, it was not the traumatic ending of a 20-year relationship, not even the loss of my health. The most detrimental death of all was in fact the unacknowledged, silent and drawn-out death of the Self. It was the gradual process of disconnection that had crept in like the slow spread of bindweed, entwining its reach all the way to my soul — suffocating my joy, my health and my heart.

For years I carried the assumption that a huge part of me had died alongside my family. It was only when truly connecting with my life story through the wisdom of my intuitive-Self that I realized this deathly destruction had in fact spread out from those first childhood moments of Self-abandonment.

As a young girl, I would often tell my parents of future events that would unfold if particular decisions were made. I'd see illness in strangers and mention a vortex of warm swirling energy in my hands and fingers, but no one around me had any idea of what this meant, so this was shut down too. At the age of seven, after my granddad died, I told my mum that my uncle, her younger brother, would die of a broken heart. It turned out he did have heart issues; in fact, unbeknownst to me, he was waiting for a triple heart bypass. He died of heart failure that same year.

I had a pretty strong knack for knowing about births too. I remember my mum scolding me after a visit to my aunt's house when I spoke of a blonde girl, Sally-Anne, waiting to be born. In fact, I explained, there were two girls, both with blonde hair. I didn't know my aunt had been having trouble conceiving – until she had two blonde daughters, one called Sally and the other Annie.

All of these 'knowings' felt normal to me, no different from anything else I might know, but whenever I spoke out about them, I was shut down in one way or another. By the age of nine or ten, I shut them down from the inside too. Often, as I lay between the worlds of sleep and wakefulness, 'otherworldly' sounds, visions and sensations would haunt me – and I'd be terrified! Somehow the energy of that fear was just the right ingredient to close down my access to this unexplained world for many years to come.

It was that disconnection from my authentic Self, that denial of my spiritual truth, of all I was and all I was meant to become, that lay beneath the years of repeated chronic illness and debilitation. It took many years for me to acknowledge that this was my body expressing the pain of my truth. I had belittled my intuition, ignored my gut, shut down my heart, discounted my thoughts and disallowed my feelings, so much so that each and every time I strayed too far out of alignment, my body would fight for reconnection and unity, shouting *so loudly* that I had no choice but to listen. If I wanted to live a life free from suffering, I was left with no choice but to repair and reconnect with all those abandoned levels of the Self – body, heart, mind and soul.

A DISCONNECTED SELF ACROSS YOUR LIFE

Disconnection and the resulting difficulties not only impact us on all our levels of the Self but they also impact our timeline – a line running from before our birth to the current moment and on into the future. We need an awareness of our past to learn from it and a view of the future so we can work towards it, but we must also remain connected and attentive to living in the now. As such, we must check in with the Self and use strategies to balance and connect with *all* the levels of our existence across all of time.

How often do you allow yourself the gift of living in the present moment, fully engaging with and experiencing your life and all it brings? How able are you to truly *feel* into your lived experience in the now? Just think about that for a moment. Are you *really* present, or has life, present or past, led you to disconnect from this also?

Many of us unwittingly tend to reside in the past or in the future, spending our time thinking and feeling into a rerun of times gone by or anticipating what's to come next, most often through a lens of fear and worry. Take note of where your thinking tends to habitually gravitate, as the further you are from the now, the further you are from the Self, and from those conscious changes that can lead you to a fulfilling future.

Connecting with Your Timeline

Close your eyes, take a deep breath and allow your focus to drop into the body.

Pay immediate attention to your first response when I give you the next instruction. It's your intuitive mind that has the answer, not your logical mind.

Just assume your timeline is a line running from your past to your future. If I say, 'Point to your past,' where is it?

How about your future? Where is that?

And what about your present? Does the line connecting the past with the future go through the body or is it somewhere outside of you?

///

This is a strange concept, I know, yet when working with clients and asking these questions, I've found they have an instinctive awareness of their timeline. Upon reflection, how it's conceptualized in their mind can often be seen as a metaphorical or symbolic representation of how their lives are playing out in the present.

For example, where do you habitually store your past? Behind you, in front of you, to the left or to the right? Perhaps even below you? Just imagine for a moment the impact that placement might have on your life. If your past is unconsciously stored in front of you, on some level you're constantly faced with it. That might be okay if you believe you can use knowledge from past experiences to move forwards and grow, but if that past is repeatedly causing distress, it'll no doubt detrimentally interfere with your daily life. I have seen this with clients who are overly involved in or influenced by their past. Either it is directly in front of them and their future behind them, or it is laid out in front of them from left to right, or right to left. No wonder it's hard to let go and move forwards.

If the future is metaphorically out of sight, this also explains why people struggle to move towards it. Again, I often see this in clients living in survival mode, just getting through life day by day, with no clear direction. Future possibilities don't exist, as they aren't consciously visible. From this perspective, it's easy to become stuck, depressed and disillusioned.

It is better to consciously reorient your timeline and store the past behind you, so you can focus on the present and the future. Knowing how to influence your timeline can be really helpful when reviewing your past and generating a future life you wish to live. We will be doing this at various points in the book. For now, you can see some timeline examples in the diagram below:

—— Main timeline running through the body. Present is in the body.
- - - - Timeline disconnected from the body. Present is outside of the body.
—— Timeline running through the body diagonally. Present is in the body.

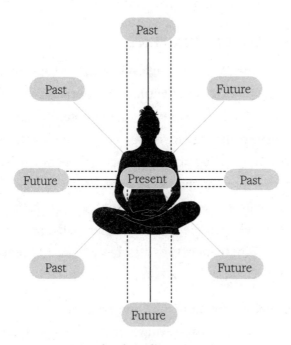

Examples of Timeline Orientation

As can be seen from the diagram, when people are more present and consciously connected to their lives, their timeline passes through their body, regardless of where their past and future are located. In some instances, though, often when a person is totally disconnected from their life, their line passes in front of, behind or next to their body, so they are a mere observer in their life rather than a participant. I see this more often when someone has had some kind of trauma or is experiencing depression or is grieving.

Front to back, back to front timelines are the most common, but I also sometimes see timelines running diagonally. This has pretty much the same meaning – either you can't fully let go of the past or fully commit to the future. One foot in, one foot out!

Timelines can be extremely revealing. I have seen down timelines my whole life, which is why I can often predict what's likely to happen in the future if someone takes a particular course of action.

DISCONNECTED DISCONTENT

Are you ready now to take a new course of action? Perhaps you're more aware of the disconnect you carry from within the separate layers of the Self. You might even have gained an awareness of a disconnect from your timeline too. Perhaps you've realized that you so overly identify with your past, that you're often trapped feeding hungry ghosts, or that you're so preoccupied firefighting in your present that there's just no possibility of flirting with your future. Or maybe you're so connected to your future dreams that you've lost all grounding in the lived experience of the present moment and with no action to fulfil them in the now, they will forever remain just that – unfulfilled dreams!

Disconnection looks different to each and every one of us and is outwardly expressed in its own unique way. However it is expressed, though, no level of the Self remains untouched, which is why we're now in need of a more integrated approach to health and healing. We need science to evolve more fully and to move beyond the confines of the medical model, where illness relates to an isolated organ of a separate body and mind, and the energetic body (and our influence over it) is reduced to a figment of our imagination.

One of the drawbacks of the modern-day world we live in is that our education systems exclude higher-frequency energy, consciousness or spirit, from the curriculum, resulting in an incomplete understanding of the nature of life and the mechanics that underpin reality.

This fracture between the spiritual and physical most probably originated with the scientific revolution, when science began identifying only with the material and anything relating to the spirit was split off and placed within religion. The age of scientific materialism, and its associated teachings, has almost certainly led to this disconnection from the spiritual/energetic layer of our being, and as a consequence, the loss of knowing all that we are and all that we're capable of achieving.

Fortunately, when fully connected, one of the many things we're capable of achieving is healing.

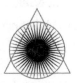

CHAPTER 4

WELLNESS IS AN INSIDE JOB

We all have innate healing potential within us. It lies dormant, a patient teacher, just waiting for the right circumstances for its discovery. We can all intuitively perceive what we need for our mental, physical, emotional and spiritual healing. The biggest challenge for most of us is learning to listen to the language of our body and to trust in this inner guidance. But I *know* this can lead to recovery.

'Spontaneous recovery??!!!'

These were the words the endocrinologist added to my hospital notes, written in large biro letters across the centre of the page. There was nothing more he could say. My recovery didn't fit the theoretical assumptions and outcome measures he'd expected from his experience and training in the medical model. It didn't meet any of his expectations whatsoever!

I had stepped into Dr Baxter's office with immense trepidation that day. He'd wanted me to restart my medication for nearly a year, and I'd managed to drag it out, persuading him at each consultation to wait just that little bit longer, but I knew my time was running out. During our last appointment, I had promised I would discuss going back on my tablets at our next meeting. My levels of prolactin were getting higher and higher and my symptoms were growing in intensity day by day, with near-constant headaches, dodgy vision and a fogginess that at times betrayed my desire to display the stoic professionalism I had placed above my own basic needs.

Six weeks earlier, Andrea, an old friend of mine, had come to visit. She lived many miles away and hadn't seen me for some time. When I opened the door, she just stood and stared. Short moments later, greeting me with tears in her eyes, she confessed I looked like I was about to die!

Not quite the reunion I had expected. I liked to pretend I was okay. I was the strong one. Regardless of what was going on in my world, my smile was always waiting in the wings, next to a slice of cake and a cup of empathy. I was so used to keeping up the act, it stunned me that Andrea saw straight through to the deep pain concealed behind the façade.

I'm sure you can all relate to this. It's what I call the 'I'm okay' epidemic. As a collective, we seem to have developed the idea that we need to protect others (and often ourselves) from the bleak realities of our lived experience and that it's not socially acceptable to say how we truly feel. But sadly, by furnishing others with only that which is deemed tolerable, we disconnect from the reality of our truth and are destined to feel isolated and alone as a result.

Carl Rogers, the father of Person-centred therapy, termed this process Conditions of Worth. It's a process whereby we learn from the messages we receive in childhood that we must meet certain criteria in order for our loved ones to accept us as worthy of their love or positive regard. As our lives progress, so does this denial of the Self, until we're left with an empty vessel bearing little resemblance to the person reflected back from deep within the mirror.

Despite Andrea's response, I still had no intention of going back on the medication with the horrendous side-effects, some of which can only be described as visual hallucinations and delusional thinking. One Sunday afternoon, for example, I had to fight the intense compulsion to throw myself from the top floor of a busy shopping centre. Surely this awful medication wasn't the only way to protect myself from potential brain surgery at the tender age of 22.

I'd already been through so much. Over the preceding few years, I'd had five laparoscopic operations to laser endometriosis, and had been in and out of day wards having test upon test, including MRI scans, ultrasounds and visual field tests. I had already been given the news by two doctors, on two separate occasions, that it would be extremely unlikely I would ever have my own children, due to the pituitary tumour, endometriosis and scar damage from an operation to remove a large ovarian cyst.

It seems a strange thing to say, but despite the medical mayhem, a part of me never fully identified as the person 'suffering' from all these physical complaints – something I now know helped me to heal and to recover. Don't get me wrong, I wasn't immune to the hopelessness and helplessness, and I did suffer immense pain and terrible physical symptoms for much of the time. But running parallel to this, I had an inner knowing. I knew that this was all a part of a much bigger story, I knew from a young age I would sample much suffering, I knew I was here to help people to heal themselves and I knew that there was another way to do just that. I just didn't yet know what that would be.

COMING BACK TO THE SELF

The week after Andrea's visit, Sonya, a temp from my office at Reuters, said something that would set in motion the sequence of events leading to my journey of transformation, self-healing and spiritual awakening.

As I handed her a list of meetings to organize, she confessed, 'My husband has a strong feeling he's meant to help you...'

Long story short, I humoured her and ended up driving over to her flat a few nights that week so she and her husband, Lindsay, could do what they called Reiki healing. I was to lie on their bed and close my eyes and just relax as they waved their arms over me – this was apparently a form of healing! I was exceptionally sceptical and uncomfortable, and to be honest I wouldn't have gone if I could have got out of it without hurting their feelings.

The first session was unremarkable, and thoughts of how I could excuse myself from our next meeting poured in thick and fast. I really didn't have time for any of this, did I? But of course I dutifully obliged.

I attended the second session with the conscious intention to surrender, to just be at one with the process. Sinking down into the bed and drifting into the darkness beyond, on this occasion I found my mind's eye was suddenly met by an amazing display of purple pulsating balls of energy radiating out and into the distance. At times it felt as if more people had gathered in the room, yet the reality was there'd been barely enough space for us to squeeze in and close the door. Confusingly, their four hands would often feel like eight, and at times even felt as though they'd penetrated my physical form, yet they never even touched me. This was such a bizarre experience yet also a strangely familiar one! The energy that swirled and danced around me felt like an old friend, and somehow my mind was transported back to my childhood.

The Reiki session that day not only opened a doorway to healing, it reunited me with the energetic level of my existence, with the world my childhood Self had locked away behind a door of fear. As I peeped round that door, I reconnected with that past and remembered all those 'unusual' experiences I'd long since forgotten!

When pondering on the Reiki session later that evening, I found my intuition telling me the tumour was the physical manifestation of a blockage within my energy field, which most probably related to having barricaded this unseen world away for so many years. I instinctively knew I could heal it by raising my vibrational frequency, bringing in healing energy and programming my mind and body with a new reality – one where the tumour did not exist. I also knew this involved an acceptance of the 'unacceptable'.

I had to know more. I immersed myself in books on quantum healing, did fast-track training to become a Reiki healer, embraced meditation and developed intuitive energy work and healing visualizations that I incorporated into my daily routine.

In the weeks that followed, I fully embraced the process of doing the work to connect with and facilitate my own self-healing. By the time I had my next appointment with Dr Baxter, my prolactin levels had miraculously reduced from 15,000 to less than 10 – no medication and no operation needed!

Leaving behind a very bemused consultant, I walked out of the hospital that day prescription-free, just as I had envisioned in my meditations. I was beyond ecstatic! But I was equally shocked – I hadn't *actually* expected it to work so well! Not only was the pituitary tumour obliterated, but a simultaneous healing of the endometriosis had also occurred and, contrary to previous professional predictions, I have two beautiful, amazing daughters today!

So, even medical doctors, with their sophisticated tests, can't always find the source of, or the resolution to, our health issues. But there is one authority that always has the answers, and that authority is within us! We can become our own best healers.

THE MIND–BODY–SOUL CONNECTION

There are parts of us that know the language of our body and all its needs, but we can't possibly attend to them if we aren't consciously present to this inner world. If we are focusing on our job, our bank balance or our next big challenge, then how can we hear the call of this inner tutor? How can we possibly witness and attend to that which our body is communicating, and how can we express, rather than repress, the associated emotions? We need to make a body-heart-mind-soul connection and listen to our *inner*-tuition.

Inner-Tuition

The *in*-tuitive part of the Self is the higher or wise Self that provides us with the '*inner*-tuition' or wisdom we need to navigate our life, remain healthy and connect with our true potential. It's that subtle voice of truth that whispers through our body and within our mind when we're feeling calm and centred. It's that inner knowing that guides us towards safety and away from harm, and it's also that powerful fear response or 'kick in the gut' that prompts us to take notice of the negative.

When we're disconnected from the Self, the energetic pathways that connect us to our own intuition, to the energies of others and to the databases of our collective super-computer run dry. But by stepping up and into our *inner*-tuition, we're by default generating a connection through all our energetic levels, from the lower-vibrational frequency of the solid physical body to the higher sensory frequencies, through which we can gain access to a limitless capacity for growth and healing for our Self and others.

The Energy Body

Each of us is an energetic being in a biological body in a physical world, so everything underpinning our current reality – environment, lifestyle, culture, personal/collective/generational trauma, genetics, epigenetics, even our thoughts – comprises an energetic blueprint from which we unconsciously live our life and relate with others. This is our *energy body*, and in order to access and fully heal on *all* levels, we need to dig a little deeper and look beyond traditional psychology so we can incorporate this energy body into the work.

One of the most important lessons I've learnt in my psychology practice and in my own life experience is that by viewing ourselves merely through a psychological or physical lens, we're impeding our chances of fully healing. If we're not looking at the energy body in tandem with the physical and the psychological, we aren't getting to the root of the problem, and if we aren't getting to the root of the problem, we'll remain stuck in a cycle of disconnected discontent, living with limited health, limited joy and limited growth.

How many times have you thought your difficulties were under control, only to have them resurface in a different way? If you're only looking at part of the problem, you're undoubtedly cutting yourself off from part of the solution.

Opening my mind and surrendering to the experience of Reiki healing expanded my conscious awareness and re-introduced me to my energy body, which ultimately led to the actions that altered the course of my life. I can therefore personally vouch for the vital role that the energy body and its vibrational frequencies play in our health and wellbeing, and yet most psychology and medical training overlooks this aspect.

There is, however, growing scientific evidence in support of the efficacy of energetic healing practices. Taking Reiki as an example, research has provided strong evidence in support of it being more effective than a placebo both for physical[1] and mental[2] health conditions. For patients with chronic health conditions, Reiki has also been found to produce results, showing a statistically significant reduction in pain[3,4] and fatigue, particularly in patient groups with cancer.[5]

It's so important for us to understand the vital role our energy body plays in our life. When viewed through the lens of quantum theory, as you now know, everything in the Universe is energy vibrating at different frequencies. This is an intricate system, interconnected at particle level and fuelled by electrical impulses. These run through us and are stored within us, so what affects one affects all.

This can be illustrated by a famous experiment in quantum science called quantum entanglement, also named 'spooky action at a distance'. In this study, scientists split an atom and sent the particles spinning in opposite directions. At a certain point, one of the particles passed through a strong magnetic field, causing its spin to change direction. According to classical physics, this should have had no effect on the other particle, which did not pass through the magnetic field. However, at the exact same moment, the spin of the other particle shifted to match that of the particle that had passed through the magnetic field, as if the two particles were still connected and in direct communication, despite the distance between them.

Experiments such as this show this universal interconnectedness and may explain how certain vibrational frequencies we're exposed to, such as traumatic or low-frequency emotions, negative thought processes or toxic environments, can detrimentally impact our health and wellbeing. If the very structure of our cells is affected by the negative energy that we're either generating, exposed to or creating blocks with, it makes sense that it could impact our tissues, organs, muscles, glands, etc., and potentially lead to illness or disease.

Interestingly, quantum entanglement could also explain how receiving a healing frequency such as Reiki could positively alter the cells in our physical body, raising our vibrational frequency to match one of flow and health. If we're to have a healthy mind and a healthy body, we require a healthy energetic field.

This philosophy forms the foundation of various healing and holistic health practices, such as sound therapy, colour therapy and electromagnetic field therapy, for example. Using optimal vibrational frequencies to release trapped energy and emotions, restore balance and promote healing in the energy field, these practices ultimately impact the health and wellbeing of the mind and the body.

As an aside, it may also explain how healing can be effectively sent to the other side of the world and how we can know things about people we haven't been told. Despite knowing this theoretically, I am often still amazed at the degree to which I am able to connect with, feel and influence another person via the internet. According to quantum entanglement, distance is irrelevant, as we're still connected, and there can also be physical or emotional entanglement between the body/mind/consciousness of two people. Both have been found in studies, like the one conducted at the University of Hawaii,[6] where functional magnetic resonance imaging (fMRI) technology captured the activation of certain brain functions at the exact time a distant healer was sending thoughts of healing intention to another person, showing, like quantum entanglement, that distance had no bearing on the connection between them.

This connection was also found in a similar experiment, where colleagues of two years who felt a connection following a 10-minute meditation[7] were placed in different rooms, one in an MRI scanner and the other in a room where they were shown a chequerboard pattern at random intervals. When the person viewed the image, the visual cortex of their colleague in the scanner was simultaneously activated, meaning that somehow this experience was shared, as both brains effectively 'saw' the image. This could provide an explanation for how I saw in my mind the exact book my client had bought just as she was thinking of it.

Without practice and presence, this energy isn't something we will typically see, feel or read. Our attention is often placed elsewhere. Yet have you ever picked up on a bad atmosphere when walking into a room? You may just *know* that moments before an argument took place there, even though you weren't present to witness it. It's as if that emotion has infected the energy of the space. Another common experience is when you're close to someone who is highly anxious, stressed or angry and you begin to feel the same, as this heavy energy radiates out, impacting everyone in its vicinity.

Interestingly, earlier this year I was at a conference where scientist and author Gregg Braden was speaking and he was discussing the electrical potential of the human body, stating that the average adult has approximately 50 trillion cells. As each cell has been measured to generate around .07 volts of electrical potential, this means, he explained, that we each have approximately 3.5 trillion volts of electrical potential available to us. Now, a typical car battery generates 12 volts of electricity, so we all have the same electrical potential as around 3 billion 12-volt car batteries. That's a lot of energy!

I'm not quite sure how accurate these calculations are in relation to the electrical potential of each individual cell, as when researching this I found some studies that quoted smaller figures. Regardless, even when taking the smaller figures into consideration, we're still looking at a vast amount of electrical potential. What if we were to harness some of that to facilitate healing ourselves or other people? Just imagine the changes we might see! And what about the rest of the energy fields that surround us? The possibilities really are unlimited.

If you're anything like me, though, you'll need your own personal experience if you're to buy into this, so let's get you in touch with your own energetic field.

Developing Your Ability to Sense Your Energetic Field

1. Take a moment to find a comfortable position, either sitting or standing, with a straight back.

2. Close your eyes and drop your awareness into the body.

3. Take three deep breaths, in through the nose and out through the mouth, making the exhale longer than the inhale.

4. Hold your hands out in front of you, palms facing each other in a praying position, and place all your attention and awareness on them for a few moments.

5. Now, bring your hands forwards so you can look at them, meaning that if still in the praying position, the fingers are now pointing forwards, perhaps to another person in front of you, instead of pointing up.

6. Now, open your hands so that there is about half an inch of space between the palms.

7. Stay focused on your hands and the space between them.

8. What do you notice? What do you feel? What changes occur?

9. What happens if you move your palms closer for a few moments? How about further apart?

10. Continue this in and out motion more quickly. What do you notice now?

11. What about if you slide your palms forwards and backwards, up and down? What does this do?

12. Open your eyes and try looking at the space between your palms.

13. Repeat the exercise. What do you see now?

14. When you feel you have explored enough, lower your hands into your lap and take three deep breaths once more.

///

Here's what to watch out for...

Most people begin noticing subtle feelings in their hands – perhaps a tingling, a change in temperature, a lightness in texture or weight. At times a stickiness may be sensed, or pressure, electrical impulses, or even a magnetic pull between the palms, especially when manipulating the energy through movement.

It's a very rare person who feels nothing when they follow these directions, but if that is you, fear not, with practice, I have absolute faith you too will consciously sense your energetic field.

Once you're more practised at this, your awareness will grow and it will be much easier to tune in to the energy. You may even see a glow around your hands or witness the movement of the energy between them. Once the invisible becomes visible, perhaps you'll notice colours, too. Eventually, you'll begin to experience a larger presence of energy and start to notice how it surrounds the body. You'll gain an awareness of the condition of your energy system too, as well as the impact of the energy coming in from other people, even from objects.

Energy Flow

This energy field, or aura, surrounding the human body is acknowledged in many healing modalities and spiritual traditions, such as Hinduism, Buddhism and Taoism. Although each has its own specific terminology and practices to describe and work with this energy, they all recognize the profound impact the energy field has in maintaining health and wellbeing.

In the same way, many ancient medical systems originating in the Far East also focus on the body's energy system, and aim to balance and harmonize the flow of energy throughout the body, mind and spirit. These include Traditional Chinese Medicine (TCM) and Ayurveda, which have been practised for around 2,000 and 5,000 years respectively. They both have a holistic approach to wellness and, unlike Western medicine, focus on the patient as a whole rather than just looking to treat symptoms or a particular disease.

Illness and disease may be biochemical or physiological in nature, but, just like everything else, also have an energetic component. When there is an irregular flow of energy in the body – when it becomes disrupted, sluggish or blocked – it impacts all the other levels of the Self and can manifest as both psychological and physiological difficulties. You see, energy is influenced by more than a terrible night's sleep, a poor diet or minimal movement. When our thoughts are inflexible and our belief system fixed, we can create a block! When we ignore our needs, fail to acknowledge our feelings or split off a part of us that we find unfavourable, we create a block!

Right now, your energetic system may very well be impacted by such mental, physical, emotional and relational blocks, as we haven't yet addressed the unwanted thoughts, feelings, impulses and/or relationships in your past. But as you move through this book, you will learn to free or move stuck emotional energy and create the space and harmony you need in your system, so you can connect with your innate healing capabilities and future life potential.

The Chakras and Meridians

Within the energy body there are various systems we can influence to facilitate transformation and healing. During the last exercise, you may have felt tiny spinning vortices of energy at the tips of your fingers or in the palms of your hands. These are chakras, spinning wheels of energy. There are seven main chakras in the body, located along the spine, from the base to the crown, each corresponding to a different vibration, colour, sound and element, as well as being associated with a different physical, emotional and spiritual aspect of the Self:

1. **Root** (*Muladhara*): Located at the base of the spine, the root chakra is associated with grounding, stability and security. Imbalance can lead to fatigue, anxieties and fear, weight gain, insecurity and poor sleep.

2. **Sacral** (*Svadhisthana*): Located in the lower abdomen, the sacral chakra represents creativity, pleasure and balanced emotions. Imbalance leads to poor creativity, isolation, withheld intimacy and sexual dysfunction.

3. **Solar plexus** (*Manipura*): Located in the upper abdomen, the solar plexus influences willpower, confidence and self-esteem. Imbalance can cause control issues, low self-esteem, manipulative tendencies and misuse of power.

4. **Heart** (*Anahata*): Located in the centre of the chest, the heart chakra influences love, compassion and emotional balance. Imbalance can lead to loneliness, depression, poor relationships, lack of discipline and resentment.

5. **Throat** (*Vishuddha*): Located in the throat, the throat chakra influences self-expression, communication and truth. Imbalance sees someone being withdrawn, shy or insensitive and having social anxiety or difficulty expressing thoughts.

6. **Third eye** (*Ajna*): Located in the centre of the forehead, the third eye chakra is associated with intuition, wisdom and spiritual insight. Imbalance presents as a lack of direction and clarity, and poor vision/memory.

7. **Crown** (*Sahasrara*): Located at the top of the head, the crown is associated with spiritual connection, higher consciousness and enlightenment. Imbalance leads to cynicism, closed-mindedness, disconnectedness and materialism.

These chakras are believed to work together to create a balanced and harmonious energy system in the body; however, if one or more of them is blocked or imbalanced, it can affect us on a mental, physical, emotional and spiritual level.

As well as different forms of energy healing, various practices such as yoga, meditation, Tai Chi and breathwork have traditionally been used to balance and activate these energy centres. Later on, we will focus on techniques that you can use to unblock, heal and transform at the energetic level of the Self. As well as the chakra system, these will relate to the meridian system – a network of 12 main energy pathways or channels through which vital energy, or *qi*, flows.

Here are the 12 meridians and what they relate to:

1. **Lung:** The lung meridian starts at the chest and runs down the arm to the thumb. It is associated with the respiratory system and helps to regulate breathing and circulation.

2. **Large intestine:** Starts at the index finger and runs up the arm to the face. It is associated with the digestive system and helps to regulate bowel movements and eliminate waste.

3. **Stomach:** The stomach meridian starts at the face and runs down the body to the foot. It is associated with the digestive system and helps to regulate digestion and appetite.

4. **Spleen:** The spleen meridian starts at the foot and runs up the leg to the chest. It is associated with the digestive system and helps to regulate digestion and the absorption of nutrients.

5. **Heart:** Starts at the chest and runs down the arm to the little finger. It is associated with the cardiovascular system and helps to regulate heart function and blood circulation.

6. **Small intestine:** This meridian starts at the little finger and runs up the arm to the face. It is associated with the digestive system and helps to absorb nutrients and eliminate waste.

7. **Bladder:** The bladder meridian starts at the face and runs down the body to the foot. It is associated with the urinary system and helps to regulate urine production and elimination.

8. **Kidney:** The kidney meridian starts at the foot and runs up the leg to the chest. It is associated with the urinary system and helps to regulate fluid balance and kidney function.

9. **Pericardium:** Starts at the chest and runs down the arm to the middle finger. It is associated with the cardiovascular system and helps to regulate heart function and blood circulation.

10. **Triple burner:** Starts at the hand and runs up the arm to the face. It is associated with the endocrine system and helps to regulate hormone production and metabolism.

11. **Gall bladder:** Starts at the face and runs down the body to the foot. It is associated with the digestive system and helps to regulate bile production and elimination.

12. **Liver:** The liver meridian starts at the foot and runs up the leg to the chest. It is associated with the digestive system and helps to regulate digestion and liver function.

Again, when the energy flowing through the meridians is blocked or disrupted, it can lead to emotional or physical imbalances, pain and illness. Each meridian has its own set of points that can be stimulated to unblock, balance or improve the flow of energy. TCM practices, such as acupuncture, acupressure, moxibustion, herbs and Tui Na massage, are techniques that are commonly used to achieve this. The meridians are believed to be interconnected, and an imbalance in one can affect the others. Therefore, TCM treatments often aim to balance and unblock the energy flow throughout the entire body to promote overall health and wellbeing.

When we have a greater awareness and understanding of both of these energy systems and do the work to restore their natural flow, alongside more traditional physiological and psychological strategies, we have a good chance of effecting real change in ourselves and the world in which we live.

Experiencing the Energy Body

To help you apply some of the healing tools in the second part of this book more effectively, I'm going to help you become more open and sensitive to the world of energy. Everything is energy and energy is everywhere – our body is energy, our emotions are energy, our thoughts are energy, even our ancestors and our future babies are energy!

Sitting in the Power

Sitting in the power will not only help you become more aware of the subtle sensations in the body and the thoughts preoccupying your mind, it will also enable you to be aware of your energy body. With practice, it can become a powerful tool to access even higher levels of consciousness.

You're developing this skill to gain a stronger awareness of your energetic field in order to build a clearer connection to your intuition and generate the foundations through which you can begin to Self-heal.

It's important you give yourself the best chance of experiencing this, so find a quiet, comfortable place where you'll remain undisturbed.

1. **Preparation**: Sit on a chair with your feet firmly planted on the ground and your hands resting comfortably in your lap. Close your eyes, take a few deep breaths to centre yourself, relax your body and quieten your mind. Send out the intention that you are going to experience your energy body.

2. **Connecting with the energy body**: Visualize roots extending down from the soles of your feet into the earth and drawing energy up into your body. Feel yourself becoming grounded and centred. Imagine a white light above your head representing divine energy and feel it flowing down into your body, filling you up with its radiance and expanding out from within you into the space around you.

3. **Merging with the energy body**: Bring awareness to the energy of your heart centre - place your hands there if it helps focus. Expand that awareness out into the space around you, just as we did with the hands. Focus on the sensations in your body and imagine this energy flowing through into the space surrounding you. Shift vibration from the physical and merge with the metaphysical.

4. **Opening awareness and insight**: Notice what changes occur in and around the body. For example, a quickening in the heart centre can feel like anxiety, but it just shows that you've connected to a higher frequency and you're vibrating slightly faster here. You may notice a movement/pulsing of energy similar to what you might have experienced in your hands. You may rhythmically move or sway, like a heartbeat, as your body is impacted by this higher frequency.

5. **Closing off and journalling**: Allow yourself to remain here, fully present to the moment, and stay open to any insights or intuitive/spiritual guidance that may come through. Then take a few deep breaths and slowly open your eyes. In your own time, journal a little on your experience. I'd recommend making the time to do this daily to deepen your spiritual awareness and connection. Be patient with yourself - developing this connection is a lifelong journey. Approach it with an open heart and a willingness to connect with your inner wisdom, and trust that with regular practice, you'll be deepening your awareness and understanding. Then a new level of information will be available to you, so you can

make more aligned choices for better health, better relationships and a better life.

If you'd like to access an extended audio version of this exercise, you'll find it on my site (*page xxvi*) and in the audiobook.

//

My hope is that this chapter has introduced you to the idea that not all healing is measurable by science alone and has helped you to embrace new potential realities. Shifting your awareness away from the analytical mind, down into the physical body and out into the energetic body, will allow you to begin to tune in to your health, your healing and your happiness more deeply.

Connections are important. It was by reconnecting to the energies I'd befriended as a child that I was able to unlock my own capacity for Self-healing. This connection would ultimately shift me onto a new timeline with a new career path, one more in alignment with who my future-Self was calling me to be. I wonder what transformations lie ahead for *you* once you've connected with your own authentic Self on all levels?

Having transformed my own health and happiness, I know that you have the power to transform your life too. So, keep reading, as I have a *whole* lot more to share with you, starting with the Release and Re-programming Method.

PART II
THE CONNECTED SELF

CHAPTER 5

THE RELEASE AND RE-PROGRAMMING METHOD

Healing is a complex process, and the journey towards becoming a fully Connected Self is unique for everyone. That's because what we carry is intrinsically linked to events encountered along our timeline, as well as the individual conditioning and programming we've acquired as a result. What's more, the way in which this message is communicated varies also, from physical illness to mental health challenges and even relationship struggles. I have developed a healing protocol that accounts for these individual differences and, if followed, can free you from your past and redirect you to a fulfilling future. It enables you to release the behaviours, emotions, thoughts and energy of what no longer serves you through each of the levels of the Self, so that you can call in the vibrational frequency of how you choose to be instead. It's called the Release and Re-programming Method.

This process comes in four stages:

1. Switching off the stress-response system
2. Gaining an awareness of past programming
3. Processing a painful past
4. Finding a fulfilling future

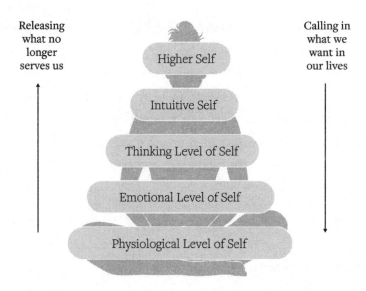

Releasing
what no
longer
serves us

Calling in
what we
want in
our lives

Higher Self

Intuitive Self

Thinking Level of Self

Emotional Level of Self

Physiological Level of Self

The Release and Re-Programming Method at each Level of Self

In this chapter we'll look at some techniques to help switch off the stress-response system – a necessary precursor to doing the work as lasting change is impossible when you're in a state of high arousal as priority is given to facing threats. First, we'll walk through a number of ways you can alter your lifestyle to start reducing the amount of stress in your bucket. You're encouraged to incorporate these strategies into your everyday life, to enable you to switch off the stress-response system, nurture a sense of safety and programme a peaceful present.

SWITCHING OFF THE STRESS-RESPONSE SYSTEM

Whether we've repeatedly faced highly stressful situations in our life, carry unresolved trauma from the past or have an insecure attachment pattern that impacts our relationship with ourselves and others, we'll remain in a state of high arousal until safety returns with the activation of the parasympathetic nervous system.

offer you some tools for switching off the stress-response
.e bring in a sense of calm and deactivation, whilst others are
those times when the demands of the world are pressing down
upo. .u and you're in immediate need of strategies to help regulate
your emotions and provide clarity of thought in the moment. This is of
paramount importance, as without it, you may not feel safe enough to work
with the tools presented in the following chapters and come home to a fully
Connected Self.

I'd like to help you to generate your own toolbox of techniques to access
in your life as and when needed. So, in your journal perhaps highlight the
strategies that resonate with your needs the most.

Worrying is the first symptom of high arousal we need to address, as worry
can generate stress and stress can then generate worry – a cycle we need to
break if we're to programme a peaceful present.

THE WORRY CYCLE

When our body's survival mechanisms are activated with no downtime to
recover, we often get pulled into a self-perpetuating cycle of worry, fear and
anxiety. The mind and body are intricately connected, as you now know,
so when in this state of high arousal, they'll go into overdrive, focusing on
'what might happen' and constantly preparing to predict and survive further
danger. But believe it or not, no matter how much time we spend dwelling
on worst-case scenarios, we're no better equipped to deal with them should
they actually happen. Instead, we're simply preventing ourselves from
enjoying what good we have in the present moment and generating the
energy that perpetuates more of the same. This creates an 'internal threat'
that our brain responds to in the same way as if the danger was actually
present in our external reality, and this can lead to incessant worry and
rumination, which, although they might start with a solvable problem, can
end in worrying about catastrophe.

This is evident in the worry chain below, which starts with the solvable worry of messing up a work presentation and ends with losing a home.

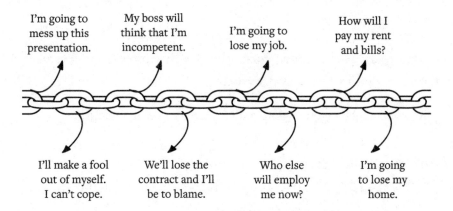

I'm going to mess up this presentation.

My boss will think that I'm incompetent.

I'm going to lose my job.

How will I pay my rent and bills?

I'll make a fool out of myself. I can't cope.

We'll lose the contract and I'll be to blame.

Who else will employ me now?

I'm going to lose my home.

Worry Chain

This is a real client example. In reality, the client just needed some presentation skills and coping strategies, yet due to his thought processing was facing the catastrophic danger of losing his home, which was clearly not a state conducive for a successful presentation.

Finding the root cause of any worry and addressing the core need is therefore of paramount importance to prevent such thinking loops occurring and to reduce the negative impact of stress on the body, mind and behaviour.

Everyone worries to some degree, and that's perfectly natural. Some thinking ahead and problem-solving can help us to plan for whatever comes our way; however, worry becomes a problem when it begins to interfere with our daily living, impacting our choices, reducing our quality of life or leaving us feeling demoralized, upset and exhausted.

Here are the differences between thinking that is an unhelpful worry and problem-solving:

Unhelpful Worry:

- Negative and repetitive thought process that becomes overwhelming.

- Detrimentally impacts mental health and interferes with day-to-day living.

- Creates a chain of thoughts and images that progress in increasingly catastrophic and unlikely directions.

- Remains stuck in a loop and you're unable to see a way out.

Problem-Solving:

- Constructive thought process focused on the flexibility to resolve problems and address the core need.

- Promotes optimism as you can devise a clear plan to tackle a problem and move forward.

- Accesses the logical thinking mind and lets go of the emotion that traps you in the worry cycle.

- Solution-focused skill, enhancing autonomy and self-esteem.

If your worrying is becoming excessive and taking over your life, for example if you've moved towards anxiety, you're avoiding things, obsessively thinking, feel compelled to behave in a certain way to cope or are struggling to sleep, it's time to work on reducing your stress levels, limiting the time spent worrying and improving your wellbeing.

WAVE THE WORRY GOODBYE

Step 1: Generating Worry Time

It may sound counter-intuitive, but scheduling 'worry time', known as stimulus control training, teaches you to contain worry to a designated time period, thereby freeing up your mind for more interesting, fun or peaceful activities in the moment. Many chronic worriers believe they can't control their thoughts and are often plagued by worry, as it spills into each and every moment of the day. Research shows, however, that through practice we can actually learn to control how often and when we worry.[1,2]

Remember, whatever we habitually do over and over again gets wired into our brain and we get better at it. So if we worry at random intervals throughout the day, our ability to worry will grow stronger. Alternatively, if we consciously choose to limit the frequency and energy invested in worry, by postponing it to be addressed at a predetermined time later that day, the worry habit starts to diminish and new neurological pathways take precedence.

Changing a habit like chronic worrying needs a repetitive, systematic approach. Simply telling yourself to stop doesn't cut it! Employing the technique below discharges anxiety and consciously retrains the mind and body to a less threatening way of being. If you wake in the night with anxious thoughts, or have worries that distract you from engaging in your work each day, this strategy is for you.

This is the process:

1. **Preparation**: Decide when your worry time will be, for what duration and in what location.

2. **Postponement**: Capture and write down your worries throughout the day and postpone thinking about them until worry time.

3. **Refocus**: Redirect attention and become mindful of the present moment using your five senses.

4. **Worry time**: Use this predetermined time to reflect on your worries and employ problem-solving strategies if appropriate.

Worry Time

You first need to decide on when you'll schedule around 20 minutes of worry time and try to stick to the same set time and place each day. This is to build a trusted routine and reinforce it as a new habit.

Then every time you catch an anxious thought, you need to delay it. Write it down for later and tell yourself, 'That's for worry time.'

Once you've captured the worry, take a deep breath, redirect your attention and refocus on the present moment, using all of your senses, and then be sure to use your pre-planned worry time later that day to address what's come up.

Remember, for this to work you must then take that time to focus on your worries and stick within your time limit. You can reconvene the following day for anything unresolved.

Even if you don't think you have anything to worry about one day, use the time for journalling anyway, as you're building in a habit and need this repetition to induce trust for when life gets tough once again.

When you set aside a specific time to consciously attend to your worries, they will gradually pop up during the containment of worry time rather than randomly throughout the day. This makes it easier for you to refocus your attention to the present moment and prevents repetitive cycles of rumination.

Step 2: Classifying Your Worry

Now, what you do with your worry time is also of great importance, so I'll provide you with a framework to aid you. The first step is to understand what form your worry takes.

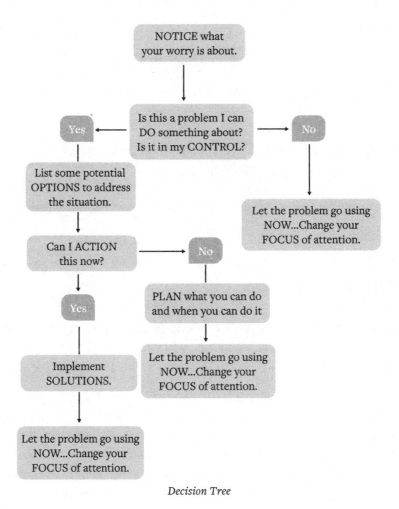

Decision Tree

Observer Stance:

- Become the observer of your worries and separate yourself from them.

- Allow your worries to be, without attempting to change or solve them.

- Accepting your thoughts and emotions can soften mental chatter and reduce suffering and worry.

- Doing all the above allows you to consciously choose a considered response, rather than impulsively reacting to situations.

Wise Mind:

- Shift your focus to a positive frequency above the worry.

- Remember a situation you've overcome or 'sit in the power' for a few moments.

- Release any attachment to a specific outcome and acknowledge that worry is just signalling you to find balance.

- Reorient yourself to address what you're *really* needing and practice self-care.

- Remember that you are safe and don't need to control anything or anyone.

You're now free to address your solvable productive worry during worry time and decide what to do about it, when to do it, how to it and actively schedule when it will be resolved. Here are some problem-solving tips to help you do this.

Step 4: Problem-solving

Worry time becomes problem-solving time when you're working with productive worry. Problem-solving involves evaluating a situation, developing concrete steps to deal with it, and then putting that plan into action.

Here you can start brainstorming multiple solutions to gain flexibility of mind and generate numerous possible outcomes for assessment. Be as creative as you like! Once you have reviewed the advantages and disadvantages of a number of solutions, you can then select one, create a plan of action, execute it and move on – free from the chains of that worrisome thought.

Before we take a closer look at these interventions, though, let's first examine a specific problem associated with stress-response activation.

Emotional Dysregulation

Emotional dysregulation refers to the difficulty in managing emotions in a healthy and adaptive way. Our ability to regulate emotions is influenced by biochemical and neurological processes associated with stress-response activation following trauma, abuse or neglect, but this is only part of the issue. Emotional dysregulation can also be specifically related to whether our emotions were responded to, validated or explained by a caregiver when we were a child. If not, the connectivity between the amygdala (responsible for emotions, survival and instinct) and the prefrontal cortex (responsible for higher cognitive functions, including emotional regulation) may be underdeveloped, and so dysregulation can remain into adulthood.

Learning strategies to improve this is a key component in finding peace in the present, processing the past and constructing a fulfilling future.

Here are some signs you may be emotionally dysregulated:

- intense/frequent mood swings

- difficulty managing stress

- impulsivity – reacting to emotions/ignoring consequences

- poor tolerance for frustration

- aggression/violent outbursts

- self-harm/suicidal ideation

- intense fear of abandonment/rejection

- difficulty maintaining stable relationships

- intense, unstable or unpredictable emotions

- avoidance/numbing behaviours, for example substance use, overeating and oversleeping

This can look like:

- a driver who gets cut off, then tails the other car for several miles in a rage of anger

- storming out of a bar when your partner catches someone else's eye

- excessively drinking alcohol to subdue nerves when meeting work colleagues

- self-harming or holding resentment when a friend cancels meeting up

Emotional dysregulation can clearly cause difficulties in many areas of life and is a key component of numerous mental health conditions, yet it is actually something we're able to influence. I'll therefore spend time explaining the science behind why breathwork in particular is so valuable and give you some examples to use for yourself.

BREATHWORK

While we can't directly access and influence the autonomic functioning of our body, our breath does so indirectly. I can't emphasize enough the impact breathwork can have on both your mental and physical health, allowing you to manage stress effectively and maintain a sense of balance and wellbeing.

How Breathwork Reduces the Stress Response

How does it work? By regulating the respiratory system, which is connected to the ANS, breathwork allows electrical signals to be sent to the brain through the vagus nerve, initiating a cascade of physiological and chemical responses that promote relaxation and reduce stress.

The vagus nerve is a complex cranial nerve running from the brainstem through the neck and down the chest and abdomen. It plays a vital role in regulating the ANS and relaying sensory information from various organs up to the brain. Interestingly, it's been suggested that approximately 80 per cent of the vagus nerve fibres send information up to the brain, while just 20 per cent run from the brain to body. This is why breathwork, bodywork, movement and somatic experiencing can be so effective at easing physiological and emotional dysregulation following stress and trauma. It also explains why talk therapy might benefit from incorporating techniques that directly impact the body – and you guessed it, this isn't usually taught during psychotherapeutic training.

So, signals from the vagus nerve help to switch off the stress-response system, enabling activation of the parasympathetic nervous system (PNS) and effectively reversing symptoms triggered by chronic stress. In Polyvagal Theory, this is termed the Ventral Vagal state and is characterized by safety, connection and engagement in social interactions. This environment is necessary to process and release difficulties and to initiate healing on all levels of the Self and within relationships.

By becoming aware of your breath and adjusting your breathing patterns accordingly, you have at your disposal a simple and really effective way to influence the quality of your life, regulate your emotions and access an inner confidence and sense of ease. You're no longer at the mercy of the body – you have the power to generate change!

Specific breathing techniques enable the activation of different branches of the autonomic nervous system, promoting either relaxation or arousal. For example, slow, deep breathing activates the PNS, promoting relaxation and reducing stress, so enabling you to have that job interview or face that phobia without becoming overwhelmed. Rapid breathing, on the other hand, activates the SNS, increasing alertness and arousal, so empowering performance during competitive events and helping you respond quickly to danger.

Reflecting on that, I'm sure you see the powerful improvements there can be for both mental and physical health when incorporating breathwork strategies in your life. Breathwork has certainly become more popular in recent years, with advocates such as Wim Hof bringing media attention to it. Not only are people becoming more inquisitive and aware of the different types of breathwork and how to utilize them to enhance performance or to heal their mind and body, but there is also now a body of research emerging to back up the benefits.

The Science Behind the Breath

There has long been anecdotal evidence to indicate an improvement in mental health conditions when incorporating breathwork in treatment, but it's also becoming more evident in the research literature. A recent meta-analysis[4] compared breathwork to non-breathwork controls from 12 randomized controlled trials and found improvements in stress, anxiety and depressive symptoms. Dysregulated breathing is a hallmark of anxiety disorders and chronic stress,[5] so it makes sense that breathwork interventions improve those symptoms. However, it's also important to note that the irregular, shallow and restricted breathing present in depression is also evidenced. What may be of interest to you is that symptoms of anxiety and depression have also been found to improve in individuals with a history of trauma,[6] and even in individuals with PTSD,[7] so do take this approach seriously, as it just might be the light at the end of a very long tunnel of sucking up unresolved symptoms.

Studies also show that breathwork has a positive impact on cardiovascular health, reducing blood pressure and heart rate,[8] and even improving heart rate variability (HRV) in people with hypertension.[9] An improvement in HRV refers to an increase in the variation of time between heartbeats. A higher HRV indicates the autonomic nervous system (ANS) is functioning well, leading to a lower risk of cardiovascular disease, improved immune function and better mental health. Conversely, lower HRV relates to health problems like chronic stress, anxiety and depression, and heightened risk of cardiovascular disease.

By shifting our breath, we influence carbon dioxide and oxygen levels, altering blood pH, which impacts cell and organ function. An overly acidic environment, for example, is linked to inflammation, immune dysfunction and other health issues. So, through simply regulating blood pH and increasing oxygenation, breathwork not only alleviates stress, it also promotes overall health and wellbeing, improving cardiovascular health, immune function, healing, brain function, circulation, energy and endurance, and reducing fatigue symptoms.

Who'd have thought the simple act of conscious breathing could impact our lives so massively?! But it doesn't stop there. Some breathwork techniques extend beyond this and work with the energy systems, whilst others foster spiritual connection or release stored trauma.

As someone with significant trauma, I've experienced the transformative power of breathwork, which can be intense, so if you too carry trauma, consult with a trauma-informed breathwork practitioner instead of attempting deeper practices alone. To ensure your safety and wellbeing, this book will prioritize breathwork for deactivating the stress response and regulating emotions, rather than processing trauma.

Experiment with the exercises below to find what works best for you and your body. Remember, breathwork accesses and changes your nervous system, so pay attention to what's happening in the body and end the practice if you begin to feel dizzy or nauseous. Focusing on the breath and body can also incite anxiety for some, so gradual exposure is key here, as is practising throughout the day when feeling calm.

Finally, use caution when holding your breath if you have high blood pressure, and if you have a respiratory condition such as asthma, alternate nostril breathing may not be for you.

Breathwork

Preparation

Before using any self-help tools, drop out of your mind and into the body to gain awareness of what is present. This will enable you to register what has changed later. Remember, everyone's body and life circumstances vary, so what works for one person may not for another.

To begin, notice how the body feels, what sensations you are experiencing and how you're breathing. Observe the pace, depth and location of your breath – is it fast or slow, deep or shallow, into your chest, into your tummy, loud or quiet, through your mouth, through your nose, or both? Understanding your natural breathing pattern empowers you to make adjustments for optimal physical, mental and emotional wellbeing.

Diaphragmatic Breathing: General Stress-Buster

Also known as belly breathing, this technique uses the diaphragm muscle to fully inhale and exhale. The inhale should be deep enough to expand your tummy, rather than just filling your chest, which is characteristic of breaths elicited by anxiety, stress and fear. Use this technique regularly to help reduce stress levels.

1. Sit/lie down, placing one hand on your belly and the other on your chest.

2. Inhale slowly and deeply through your nose, placing your awareness on breathing into your tummy.

3. Keeping your chest still, notice your hand rising as air inflates your tummy on the inhale. If your shoulders move, you're chest breathing, so keep practising.

4. Exhale slowly through your mouth, feeling your tummy deflate.

5. Repeat for several minutes.

6. Notice what has shifted in the body.

7. Repeat throughout the day to regulate oxygen levels and induce a sense of calm.

The Physiological Sigh: Immediate Regulator

This breathing pattern immediately helps discharge nervous energy for real-time stress relief.

1. Take two back-to-back inhales through the nose followed by an extended exhale through the mouth.

2. Notice the sense of relief as the body lets go of tension.

Tip: Inhale deeply, then sneak in extra air at the very end before finishing with an extra-long exhale.

The effectiveness of this technique lies in the dual inhalation, which causes the alveoli in the lungs to open, rapidly increasing oxygen intake. The long exhale then expels the carbon dioxide that builds up following emotional dysregulation, helping to rebalance oxygen levels. This is why we can often instinctively breathe this way during moments of distress.

Box Breathing: Mind and Body Balancer

Also known as square breathing, this technique calms both body and mind by synchronizing the breath and mental focus. It aids stress management, enhances cognitive function, promotes better sleep and is associated with a reduction in anxiety and depression.

1. Beginning on the inhale, place your awareness in the body and slowly exhale *all* air out of your lungs.

2. Inhale slowly through your nose for a specific count (four usually works well), saying the numbers in your mind.

3. *Hold* your breath for the same count and notice that your lungs are full of air. If holding your breath provokes anxiety, then gradually build up over time.

4. *Exhale* through your mouth for the same count and notice your breath moving up through the body and being expelled in front of you.

5. *Hold* your breath again for the same count.

6. *Repeat* for several minutes. You can even increase the count, if you wish.

7. *Notice* what's changed in the body, the mind and your energy.

Alternate Nostril Breathing: Connecting Mind-Body-Soul

This traditional yogic breath aims to align the chakra system, resulting in an interconnectedness of body, mind and soul. Channelling your breath whilst alternately closing each nostril is said to balance the left and right hemispheres of the brain. Each nostril is believed to impact emotions differently – the left affecting the feminine nurturing presence (Ida) and the right the masculine (Pingala).

Channelling the breath through each hemisphere impacts mood, as it's believed that when one side becomes weaker, the other dominates. Imbalanced left dominance is said to cause passivity and depression, while excessive right masculine energy leads to over-assertiveness. The goal is to achieve regulation and balance.

1. Sit comfortably, place your left hand on your left knee and centre your awareness on the body and breath.

2. Close your mouth and breathe exclusively through your nose.

3. Using your right thumb to close your right nostril, inhale deeply through your left nostril, expanding your ribs outward.

4. At the peak of the inhale, use the index and middle finger of your right hand to close your left nostril, releasing your right thumb.

5. Exhale through your right nostril and pause naturally at the end.

6. Inhale slowly and deeply through your right nostril, then switch and exhale through your left nostril.

7. Repeat for several minutes, gradually lengthening the exhales.

8. Notice any changes in your mind and body.

//

Be patient, as it can take time to build breathwork practices. At the very least, always breathe into your stomach and remember that lengthening the exhale slows the heart rate, generating calm, while emphasizing the inhale, whether by making it more vigorous or longer than the exhale, speeds up the heart rate, preparing you for action.

MINDFULNESS

How often do you bring yourself back to the present moment? In our fast-paced society, taking the time to be mindful is needed more than ever before.

So what is mindfulness? It was defined by Jon Kabat-Zinn, the founder of the highly regarded Mindfulness-Based Stress Reduction (MBSR) programme, as 'paying attention in a particular way: on purpose, in the present moment, and non-judgementally'.[10] It has been hailed as an effective treatment for a variety of physical[11] and mental health problems, in particular for reducing stress, anxiety and depression,[12,13] but is also consistently effective in groups of people with conditions such as chronic pain and addictions.[14] It's even been shown to boost the immune system.[15] There has been much research using the structured MBSR and Mindfulness-Based Cognitive Therapy (MBCT) programmes, which are eight-week therapeutic group programmes that combine either stress-reduction or cognitive behavioural techniques with mindfulness. Both programmes have yielded fantastic results in many of the areas researched, with MBCT specifically shown to reduce relapse in people that have experienced a major depressive episode.[16] Again, like breathwork, mindfulness is a relatively simple approach to adopt, yet it can have far-reaching positive consequences.

Recent research has shown that even just the simple mindfulness practice of paying attention to your breath can lead to improvements in your ability to regulate your emotions and improve wellbeing.[17] This is due to the increased connectivity in the brain between the amygdala and the prefrontal cortex, resulting in better integration and processing of emotional information and more effective control of emotional responses.

I shall therefore teach you a simple mindfulness exercise that you can use both as a daily tool to regulate your general stress levels and as a strategy to help in difficult moments, when it will enable you to pause and gain a compassionate sense of perspective and grounding.

A Mindful Breathing Space

This three-minute breathing space is adapted from a part of the MBCT programme.[18] It will help you to regulate and recentre yourself when your thoughts and feelings threaten to spiral out of control. To help you to easily remember the steps, I have created it as an ABC model: *Acknowledgement* of your inner experience; a narrow focus on your *Breath*; *Conscious* expansion back out to the body and beyond.

A: Acknowledgement of Your Inner Experience

Find yourself a comfortable position, whether sitting or standing, keeping an upright posture with a straight spine and neck and your feet on the ground. If possible, take a moment to close your eyes, bring your awareness to your inner experience and acknowledge what's happening for you in the present moment, asking:

1. 'What's happening in my inner experience right now?'

2. 'What *thoughts* are around?' Simply acknowledge those thoughts as mental events – the mind is doing what the mind does. Allow those thoughts to be there. You can give them a label, but choose to stay disengaged.

3. 'What *feelings* are here?' Don't try to change anything, just be open to what's already there. Taking a moment to turn towards any sense of discomfort or unpleasant feelings, notice and acknowledge them without trying to change them or make them different from how you found them.

4. 'What *bodily sensations* are here right now?' Take a moment to scan the body and notice any tension, pain or sensations of bracing. Acknowledge what you find, but once again, don't try to change it in any way.

5. 'What *energy* is here right now?' Take a moment to expand out from the body and place your awareness into the energy field around you. Notice how it moves, how it feels, what it's communicating. Acknowledge this and allow it to be just as it is right now.

B: Breath

Now it's time to gather your attention and refocus your awareness on the narrow 'spotlight' of the breath. Simply pay attention to the physical sensations of the breath, and when your mind wanders (which it will), bring your attention back to the breath each time.

1. Gently gather your awareness into the area of your abdomen, tuning in to the physical sensations of the breath.

2. Notice your abdomen expanding as the breath comes in... and falling back as it leaves the body.

3. Attend to the breath as it moves all the way down the body on the inhale and moves back up on the exhale, noticing how it feels as air passes through your nostrils, that slightly warmer temperature as it leaves the body and cooler temperature upon entry.

4. And if your mind wanders, simply acknowledge where it went and gently escort it back to the breath.

5. Use each breath as an opportunity to anchor your mind to the present moment.

6.   Remain in this space for at least five full breaths.

C: Conscious Expansion

Now, in this third and final step, we're expanding back out - opening to the field of awareness around the breath. This includes a sense of the body as a whole - your posture, facial expression, positioning in the room and energy body. In this step, you're opening to life as it is, preparing yourself for the next moments of your day.

1.   Expand your awareness out from your abdomen and open to the body as a whole, as if your whole body was breathing.

2.   Come home to the body… come home to *this* moment.

3.   Notice your posture, your facial expression, the sensations on your skin and inside the body… just as they are.

4.   Holding an awareness of all the sensations in the body right now, invite in your breath and let it soften any discomfort or tension. You're exploring the sensations and befriending them, rather than trying to change them in any way. Bringing your focus of attention into the intensity, imagine the breath moving into and around the sensations.

5.   Sit, tuning in to an awareness of your whole body *and* your energy body, moment by moment.

6.   Notice the environment around you. What sounds can you hear? What can you smell? Feel the chair, the bed or the ground beneath you.

7.   Bring this awareness with you, just as it is, as you step into the next moment of your day.

Ideally, this would be a daily practice, so it's helpful to set aside a regular time for it. You could set a reminder on your phone for every few hours, if you want to do it more than once, or, to make it a part of your daily routine, habit stack it with something else you do each day, such as brushing your teeth.

You can also listen to an audio version of this exercise. You'll find it on my site (*page xxvi*) and in the audiobook. Then, you can guide your own practice, ensuring you keep to the three-step process – beginning with an expanded attention and awareness of the physical and energetic body, zooming into a narrowed focus on the breath and then expanding back out again.

COLD THERAPY

It turns out cold water exposure, even if it's only splashing your face, is another quick and simple tool that can activate the vagus nerve, slowing down your breathing and heart rate, reducing the levels of the stress hormones cortisol and adrenaline, and promoting relaxation. Cold water exposure has also been found to increase the production of mood-elevating and pain-reducing hormones and neurotransmitters such as beta-endorphins, noradrenaline and dopamine.[19]

Now it's not for everyone, but plunging into the cold acts as a short-lived physiological stressor, which is thought to switch off the stress-response system through stimulating the body's natural survival response, known as the diving reflex. When exposed to cold water or cold air, the body will activate this reflex to slow down the heart rate and constrict blood vessels to conserve energy and oxygen, diverting nutrient-rich oxygenated blood to the vital organs such as the brain and heart.

Until recently, cold therapy was only associated with exercise recovery, pain relief and inflammation reduction, yet there is more and more research showing it to be a really great technique for reducing stress and improving symptoms in a number of mental health disorders,[20] such as depression[21] and anxiety, as well as PTSD and chronic fatigue syndrome (CFS),[22] especially when combined with static stretching[23] exercises.

Cold therapy may also be helpful if you're someone who experiences symptoms of dissociation or numbness. The shock of cold water or air can be a powerful sensory experience that can help bring you back into the body. It's becoming very popular at the moment, with people immersing themselves in ice baths on social media for all to see, but I must stress that cold therapy should not be used as a substitute for trauma-focused therapy, or other appropriate treatments for trauma-related symptoms, although under professional supervision, it can be one tool in a comprehensive treatment plan for trauma.

We all have our own individual responses to cold therapy, and some may not find it beneficial or even experience negative side-effects, so as with anything you introduce, it's important to listen to the body and your *inner*-tuition.

If you're interested in trying some cold therapy to reduce your stress activation, you could look to the Wim Hof Method,[24] which utilizes breathing techniques with cold therapy, and has been suggested to help reduce the symptoms of autoimmune conditions, PTSD and sleep disorders, to name but a few.

You can also try a few simple methods yourself:

- **Cold showers**: Start with a warm shower and gradually decrease the temperature to cold. Stay under the cold water for a few minutes before switching back to warm.

- **Cold water swimming**: Find a cold lake or ocean and take a dip. Make sure to start slowly and gradually increase the duration of your swims.

- **Cryotherapy**: This involves standing in a chamber filled with cold air for a few minutes. There are more and more venues popping up offering this service, so check out your local area.

- **Ice baths**: Fill your bath or a tub with cold water and acclimatize to the cold before you begin the process of immersion. Immerse yourself in the water for a few minutes before getting out. Your body will begin to tolerate the cold and over time you'll be able to last longer. There doesn't seem to be a universal guideline for time and temperature, but some studies seem to suggest 10–15°C water for 5–15 mins to be most effective.

It's important to note that cold therapy may not be appropriate for everyone, particularly those with certain medical conditions, so do consult your doctor first if you have heart, blood pressure or other circulatory conditions.

GROUNDING

Whilst you may have noticed a pleasant sense of calmness and wellbeing as you feel cool dewy grass beneath your feet in the garden or stroll along a warm sandy beach whilst on holiday, I suspect you might not have associated those feelings with an energetic reconnection between yourself and the Earth via a process referred to as grounding.

Grounding, or earthing, refers to direct skin contact with the surface of the Earth, such as with our bare feet and hands, or through conductive devices such as mats, bands, cords, and patches that can be used on the body, in your house or in your shoes. When a person makes direct contact with the earth in one of these ways, the electrons from the Earth's surface are believed to neutralize the positively charged free radicals in the body, which can lead to numerous health benefits.[25] A study in the *Journal of Environmental and Public Health* concluded that reconnecting with these electrons has the potential to trigger positive physiological changes and can 'strongly influence bioelectrical, bioenergetic and biochemical processes that appear to have a significant modulating effect on chronic illnesses'.[26]

These findings are confirmed by numerous other studies that have noted reduced blood viscosity, a reduction in pain and inflammation,[27] rapid wound healing, improvements in sleep, reduced stress, increased HRV and parasympathetic activation,[28] and also suggest grounding in the treatment and prevention of chronic inflammatory and autoimmune diseases,[29] as well as chronic fatigue syndrome,[30] anxiety and depression,[31] and cardiovascular disease.[32]

Some of these studies are small, but alongside the anecdotal evidence, they certainly provide a reason to incorporate grounding into your routine. It's another really simple and easy process that can aid your self-regulation and self-healing, so why not include it as an additional powerful daily practice that can help programme a peaceful present and prepare you for a happy, healthy future? I know from my own transformative experiences that when fully present to the energy of the Earth, I have literally felt the energy flowing up through me, almost as if I was plugged into a root network of energy recharging me all the way to my soul.

So, let's show you some ways you can do this for yourself. Whichever you choose, be sure to do it as a conscious mindfulness practice. Remain present, focus on your breath and really imagine connecting with nature. Feel rooted, bring in *all* your senses, including your *inner*-tuition, and notice what sensations or energy you feel as you do so.

Methods include:

- walking outside on natural ground in bare feet

- lying down on the ground and imagining connecting with your heart

- sitting on the ground, leaning up against a tree

- forest bathing – walk through a forest, feeling the earth beneath the ground and connecting with the energy from the trees

- swimming in a lake, river or ocean, or even taking a bath

- gardening, feeling the soil with your bare hands

- using grounding mats, blankets, patches, and socks

Now you have some really simple and effective scientifically backed techniques that can help you to quieten a heavily activated stress-response system. There are also many more you can incorporate into your life. If you take the body scan (*page 44*), for example, and follow the same directions but tense and release your muscles along the way, it becomes an exercise called Progressive Muscle Relaxation (PMR), which has been shown to be effective in reducing the symptoms of anxiety and improving sleep quality.[33] Body practices such as yoga[34] and Tai Chi[35] have also been found to increase heart rate variability (HRV), which, if you remember, stimulates the parasympathetic nervous system and promotes relaxation. They have also been shown to significantly reduce depression[36] and anxiety disorders, with trauma-informed yoga specifically found to help alleviate symptoms of PTSD.[37] Even massage therapy, something here in the West we often see as self-indulgent, has been shown to reduce depression and anxiety, increase attention and concentration, and aid the immune system,[38] as well as reducing occupational stress.[39]

So, now you have a fully stocked toolbox, and have been incorporating these techniques into your daily routine, you will be less physiologically aroused and psychologically preoccupied by stress, and therefore more present to begin to examine what has been troubling you.

CHAPTER 6

GAINING AN AWARENESS OF PAST PROGRAMMING

A great many people come to therapy not wishing to 'waste time' focusing on their past; they'd rather cut to the story of their life in the now and fast-forward to the happily ever after. Whilst there's nothing inherently wrong with wishing to focus on becoming a *better* version of ourselves in the now, if we do so when running on autopilot, disconnected from our past-Self, our unprocessed emotions and difficulties will simply resurface elsewhere, and we will remain destined to unconsciously project this past onto the future... again... and again... *and* again!

Have you ever wondered why all your relationships keep meeting the same fate, for example? That when you strip away the detail, the same expression of jealousy or insecurity prevails. Or maybe, despite all your best efforts to change, you keep struggling to break free from addictions, always end up broke, miss out on promotion or are always the friend that gets left behind!

It's our earliest experiences in life that form the template of who we are to become, a kind of blueprint that maps out how we see the 'realities' of this world – who we believe we are, who we believe we can become and whether we see others as friends or foes along the way. When armed with an awareness of this blueprint, we gain the power to write a new script, direct and produce each new scene, and play the starring role on a timeline of our choosing.

Dr Gabor Maté, a highly regarded trauma specialist, states that children aren't necessarily traumatized because they get hurt, they're traumatized because they're alone with that hurt.[1] I would expand on this further and state that it isn't only having no one to turn to that can increase the probability of trauma, it's the resulting abandonment and shattering of the Self that generates and exacerbates those wounds.

So, as a child, who did you turn to when you needed help, support or comfort? How did you process your pain? Express your difficulties? Who do you turn to now, as an adult? Anyone? Or do you just keep on going alone, pushing past all obstacles, soldiering on, regardless of that part of you that screams for you to stop, implores you to find help and begs you to take a break? Perhaps you're still in denial of what you are carrying, maybe even swallowing down your truth with yet another bottle of Jack – that is, until rock bottom shows up.

THE PRESENT-PAST

When we haven't had the space, time or capacity to process what's happened in our life, there is really no such thing as a 'past-Self'. We can only ever be in the present moment, so our unresolved past will be there too – right alongside us! There will be no separation between who we are now and what we experienced in the past.

Ignoring what we are carrying from the past and focusing purely on easing present pain or fantasizing over the future is like carrying an invisible backpack full of heavy rocks. Just because we can't see it and/or our focus is elsewhere doesn't mean its weight isn't pulling us down, sapping us of energy and preventing us from finding the liberation we'd unleash once released from such a hefty haul.

Like those rocks, the unaddressed wounds from the past don't simply vanish because we choose to ignore them. Instead, they embed themselves deeper into our unconscious mind and energy field, where they find expression through our thoughts, our feelings and our actions, or as blockages, creating illness in our physical body.

It's only by acknowledging and letting go of the emotional charge and mental narrative that bind such a past to our identity that we get to consciously connect with our desired future and identify with that instead. We are then free to use our future to propel us forwards, instead of allowing our past to pull us back.

THE TIMELINE OF TRANSFORMATION

The Timeline of Transformation provides the framework that will help you connect to and release past events that you may have split off from and that may be having effects you're not consciously aware of. Having switched off the stress-response system and programmed a peaceful present in chapter 5, we can now travel back to gain awareness of and process this past. We can then zoom forwards to connect with the future-Self, to shift the timeline into a new direction towards where you want your future to be and then call this into the present moment.

Examining the Past

Even before our birth we're already being moulded by the internal and external conditions we're exposed to. We may change and adapt in response to our environment, but everything we are today is rooted in all that came before. This creates a set of subconscious rules that generate the lens through which we see the world. In order to take conscious control over our destiny, we need to rewrite the pre-programmed conditioning that ties us to our past and release ourselves from the energetic hold it has over our future.

To embark on this journey, you'll need to gain a fuller picture of who has been playing the main character in your life for all these years. You'll also need to uncover what lies beneath how you see yourself, how you see others and how you see the world. Is it a safe place, or one to be feared? Do you get your needs met, by yourself and others, or do you feel the world is against you, that you're destined to be a loser in life, whilst everyone else kicks back, leisurely supping from their cups of abundance? Creating a timeline offers you the opportunity to explore how certain negative life events have affected you in the past and recognize that they may still be influencing you in the present.

An Unconsciously Pre-programmed Timeline

Once a situation becomes embedded, either through a personal encounter or through a narrative that's repeatedly shared with us, it eventually bypasses the conscious mind and evolves into an unconscious programme that, moving forwards, shapes how we perceive and engage with the world. So, when we live on autopilot, not only has our life been unconsciously programmed to a destination set by our past, but this programming inevitably becomes the driving force for future experience, keeping us stuck in a perpetual feedback loop that just keeps on giving us more and more of the same.

Living in this autopilot mode means we aren't fully present in the now, or able to make conscious decisions about how to live our lives or where we're going next. There's no way to override the old, conditioned programming by consciously creating the new, so we can only ever live according to what we already know from the past – and may never have wanted.

A Consciously Constructed Timeline

When we have reconnected with the Self, however, on every level, we're able to consciously generate a timeline in alignment with who we want to be and how we want to live.

A consciously constructed timeline occurs when there is a present awareness of and conscious connection with the past-Self. This enables acknowledgement and processing, so the past can be consciously integrated in the present, while remaining safely rooted in the past. This means unwelcome elements from that past – unprocessed emotions, suppressed thoughts, repressed memories, trauma, etc. – are no longer split off, residing in the present and being unconsciously projected onto the future.

With a consciously constructed timeline, there is also a connection with the future-Self, which is brought into the present moment so that the thoughts, feelings and behaviours of that Self can be consciously programmed into the present-Self, generating a vibrational match to that outcome. This shifts us onto this new timeline.

Let me just define what I mean by all these timeline elements to the Self:

- **Past-Self:** This is the 'memory' of you in the past as you reflect from the present moment, consisting of the time before, during and after your birth. Do note, however, that such memories have been found to be unreliable. Details change in the mind, so this is often just a story we've repeatedly told ourselves to reinforce and fit the identity of who we think we are, rather than 'fact'.

- **Past-Present-Self:** This is the Self in the past that was present at a specific time in history.

- **Future-Past-Self:** This is the potential Self in the future that has remained on unconscious autopilot, making it a version of the past-Self at a future time.

- **Present-Past-Self:** This is the Self in the present that has remained on unconscious autopilot. It's therefore just another version of the past-Self but in the present moment.

- **Present-Self:** This is the Self fully conscious to, and released from, the hold of the past. It is therefore able to be fully connected with the experience of the Self and life in the present moment.

- **Present-Future-Self:** This is the Self in the present moment that has opted to live from a future-Self perspective – proactively choosing to generate, instill and follow a programming that is specifically based on the outcome, aspirations and endless possibilities they wish to call in from the future.

- **Future-Self:** This is the Self in the future that is fully conscious to, and released from, the hold of the past.

Constructing a Timeline of Transformation is the first step to releasing what you carry from the past, but before you dive into creating your own, I'd like to introduce an example...

My client 'Fiona',* a high-achieving barrister in her early forties, presented as emotionless and cold; it was as if her soul was trapped beneath a thick wall of ice. Her posture was rigid, there was limited animation in her facial expression and she was so detached from the words she conveyed, she could have been reading from a book. Despite her stoic presentation, I felt her intense anger and deep despair, alongside a gargantuan grief that layered the walls of her prison of ice. Her world was devoid of all joy, as she had recently discovered her husband was leading a double life – even fathering other children. Reluctantly seeking therapy to salvage her marriage 'for the sake of [their] daughter', she'd deeply suppressed her emotional needs and refused to acknowledge the reality of her husband's secret family, forcing him to do the same. It was only following diagnoses of ulcerative colitis and rheumatoid arthritis, both autoimmune diseases, that she was willing to accept that the raging anger she was carrying inside was burning its way through her body.

Creating a timeline revealed for Fiona the multitude of traumatic life experiences that underpinned her perfect façade. She realized it wasn't just

---

* Names have been changed to maintain confidentiality.

this abandonment and betrayal she'd buried deep; she was also harbouring resentment about her mother's suicide when she was seven years old, her father's neglect, fuelled by his addictions, *and* his betrayal when sending her to boarding school so he could escape the pain of losing the old family by building a new one. She had then been exposed to inappropriate behaviour from her housemaster throughout her last years of school, and this was closely followed by the death of her brother, also to suicide.

Fiona discussed these events with detachment, and it became clear to me how disconnected she needed to be to survive. However, the very defence mechanisms that protected her from harm had also prevented her from healing. We can't just pick and choose which feelings to allow – if we split off from one 'unacceptable' or threatening emotion, we turn down them all. Then, devoid of all *real* feeling, we lose any enjoyment and engagement in life. The only way for Fiona to survive the reality of her situation and re-engage with life was to acknowledge her traumas and their current impact on *all* levels of the Self.

Fiona's story illustrates how a timeline has the potential to reveal to you repeated patterns within your family, and within your own thoughts and behaviours, along with helping you to join the dots between your past experiences and your present. Fiona gained an awareness of how a template for emotional suppression, abandonment, betrayal and neglect lay within her family line and her own timeline, which brought forth a deeper understanding and awareness of her current difficulties. She thought she'd come to therapy to heal her marriage, but found she needed to process and release much more! With some insight into your own timeline, you too can release the hidden burdens you are carrying from the past instead of carrying them into your future.

The Timeline of Transformation lets you observe your life from a bird's eye perspective and see the patterns or themes that have developed along the way or could develop in the future. You can then gain insight into any maladaptive thought and behavioural patterns, along with any relational re-enactments you've created in response. Becoming more conscious of the realities of the past will also provide you with the opportunity to develop compassion for yourself in the present.

This past section of the timeline is basically a list of events from your personal history. Such events can take many forms, so release any judgement and simply look at *your* life experiences and how they affected *you*. Whatever comes to mind as relevant *is* relevant; the loss of a beloved cat, for example, may affect the body and plague your mind as profoundly as the loss of a human family member. You're not here to judge your feelings; you're here to be present for yourself, to understand how events have been for *you* and to acknowledge *your* pain – perhaps for the very first time.

Creating Your Timeline: The Past-Self

Find a safe and comfortable spot in your home where you won't be disturbed. Perhaps make a nest of some soft blankets and cushions and wear some comfy clothes – it's important you set a scene of nurturance, especially if you already know there is some trauma in your past. Dim the lights and perhaps light some scented candles with a familiar smell that allows you to feel safe and calm. Play some gentle and peaceful music in the background, if that helps. Know you're safe. Know you're being looked after.

Now, I can't possibly know your history, so we need to connect with your higher Self and check out if it's okay for you to go deep now or whether it would be better for you to return to this exercise at a later date, or with some additional therapeutic support.

So just close your eyes and connect with your safe space for a moment or two, as if you're going to meditate. Take a few long, deep breaths... Let the outside world fade away and allow yourself some space... some time... just for you.

Then drop your awareness into the body...

What do you notice?

How does it feel to be *you* right now... in *this* moment?

Take a moment to quieten your mind and ask, 'Is it okay for me to access the timeline that relates to my past in order to gain an awareness of the difficult events that are contributing to my suffering in the present day?'

Take another pause...

What do you notice *now*? What's different?

Allow space for the answer and await the response – it will come.

//

Before beginning the exercise, I recommend you read it through at least once in order to familiarize yourself with it. If you've decided you're not yet ready, read it through anyway for completion at a later date. This is deep work for some, so will resonate differently for each person. Should you need to stop at any point during this or any of the following exercises, bring to mind your safe space (*see page 16*), sit with the thoughts, emotions and sensations, then imagine beaming them into your safe space container and locking them up with a key, or chains if need be – whatever feels instinctively right. Come back to the present moment, ready to continue with your day, knowing they're safely contained until you choose to reconnect another time.

I encourage you to conduct this exercise in whatever way resonates with you. You can choose to purely focus on identifying the difficult life encounters you'll be working with later, or take a balanced approach and incorporate positive experiences too. If you have a traumatic past or are currently depressed, you may find it harder to access childhood events, specifically positive ones. This is entirely normal. Give it a try anyway, as the act of engaging with it can help the memories to surface.

You'll find various timeline options in the worksheets available on my website (*page xxvi*) or you may wish to work freehand. When I'm conducting this exercise with clients, we draw a timeline from before birth to the present moment across a large white board. Use whatever feels comfortable to you.

Before beginning your Timeline of Transformation, create a Life Event Rating Table that lists major life events that occurred within a certain timespan. Place a rating next to the degree to which that event has influenced your life in the positive (+1 to +10) or the negative (–1 to –10), the higher numbers on either scale denoting a higher emotional impact.

Here's Fiona's Life Event Rating Table as an example:

Age	Positive Life Events	Rating (+)	Negative Life Events	Rating (–)
0–8	No memory of happy event	0	Stillborn sister when aged 3	6
			Mother diagnosed with M.S.	4
			Mother committed suicide	5
9–16	Made England Junior Squad	3	Dad had car accident when drunk	6
	Holiday with dad and brother	3	Sent to boarding school	7
			Dad re-married and had children	10
17–24	Academic awards and qualifications	2	First boyfriend broke her heart	6
	Ran the London Marathon	4	Sexually abused by her housemaster	4
	Went travelling and met her husband	6	Her brother committed suicide	10
25–32	Got desired pupillage	5	Had two failed IVF attempts	6
	Bought first home and got married	4	Husband's business folds	4
	Won £20,000 lottery	3	Cancer scare	5
33–43	Won high-profile court case	5	Traumatic pregnancy and birth	6
	Daughter born	3	Husband had an affair and child	8
			Diagnosed with M.E and R.A.	10

To identify events for processing later, we need to assess their emotional charge in the present. Tune in to each memory briefly and rate, out of 10, the level of emotional intensity it evokes. If a memory is too painful to access directly, it's fine to make an educated guess about its impact. Equally, if you feel no emotion, mark it as a zero. It may be you've already processed the event, so it has no emotional charge; however, it *could* be a sign of dissociation. Noticing this pattern with numerous memories may indicate emotional dissociation or repression as a core coping mechanism, pointing to a need for additional one-to-one support.

Now place these events on your past timeline, perhaps choosing to colour code certain themes for clarity, e.g., all abandonment events might be marked in blue, bereavement in black, achievements in green, etc. This will help you see patterns at a glance.

For guidance, some of Fiona's timeline is displayed on page 118 to show the repeated patterns of Abandonment, Trauma and Mental/Physical Illness prior to her birth and throughout her life.

Timeline Takeaways

As you build your own timeline, you'll identify challenges and patterns that may need attention and healing. This awareness will help you know which areas to work on with the Release and Re-programming Method and Hierarchy of Healing (*see page 153*).

For now:

Reflecting on Your Timeline

▲ What stands out on your timeline? Are there any significant observations or patterns?

▲ Which periods of your life were particularly challenging? Can you identify common themes associated with those times?

▲   What unresolved experiences need attention before you can release them - is there someone from that period you need to talk with? Something you need to do for closure? Write down what you needed *then* that you didn't have, and what you need *now* to move forwards.

▲   What painful relationship patterns from the past are still present in your life?

▲   With hindsight, what gifts did these events bring? What are the silver linings? How have these events helped you to grow as a person? If you struggle to see the silver lining, reflect on whether you could find one and consider whether this is typical of you, i.e., do you typically struggle to find a positive? Seek the support of someone else to help you find it if necessary. Many people strive to 'know why' and need to shift their thoughts, but not everyone will do so at this mental level. Yet it will be cleared later regardless.

What was it like for you to complete this task? Did you experience resistance or avoidance? Did you feel overly emotional? Did you feel numb? Were you able to find the embedded lesson or gift? Get to know yourself on a deeper level by exploring how you cope when confronting your past difficulties. Chances are you're doing something very similar in the present.

As you have seen from this chapter, you weren't born in a vacuum, and your significant relationships and the environment in which you grew up (your family, culture, religion, etc.) also need to be considered if you're to identify and understand your patterns of behaviour, relationship difficulties and even mental and physical illnesses such as depression, anxiety and addictions.

Next we'll look at how trauma can be experienced very early in life and can be passed down the generations.

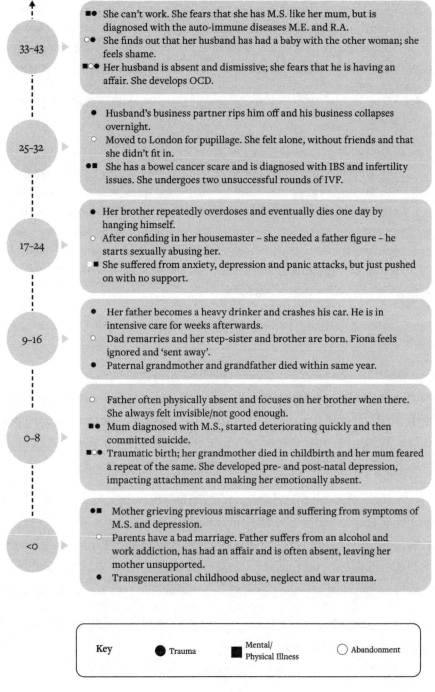

33–43
- ■● She can't work. She fears that she has M.S. like her mum, but is diagnosed with the auto-immune diseases M.E. and R.A.
- ○● She finds out that her husband has had a baby with the other woman; she feels shame.
- ■○● Her husband is absent and dismissive; she fears that he is having an affair. She develops OCD.

25–32
- ● Husband's business partner rips him off and his business collapses overnight.
- ○ Moved to London for pupillage. She felt alone, without friends and that she didn't fit in.
- ●■ She has a bowel cancer scare and is diagnosed with IBS and infertility issues. She undergoes two unsuccessful rounds of IVF.

17–24
- ● Her brother repeatedly overdoses and eventually dies one day by hanging himself.
- ○ After confiding in her housemaster – she needed a father figure – he starts sexually abusing her.
- ■ She suffered from anxiety, depression and panic attacks, but just pushed on with no support.

9–16
- ● Her father becomes a heavy drinker and crashes his car. He is in intensive care for weeks afterwards.
- ○ Dad remarries and her step-sister and brother are born. Fiona feels ignored and 'sent away'.
- ● Paternal grandmother and grandfather died within same year.

0–8
- ○ Father often physically absent and focuses on her brother when there. She always felt invisible/not good enough.
- ■● Mum diagnosed with M.S., started deteriorating quickly and then committed suicide.
- ■○● Traumatic birth; her grandmother died in childbirth and her mum feared a repeat of the same. She developed pre- and post-natal depression, impacting attachment and making her emotionally absent.

<0
- ●■ Mother grieving previous miscarriage and suffering from symptoms of M.S. and depression.
- ○ Parents have a bad marriage. Father suffers from an alcohol and work addiction, has had an affair and is often absent, leaving her mother unsupported.
- ● Transgenerational childhood abuse, neglect and war trauma.

Key	● Trauma	■ Mental/ Physical Illness	○ Abandonment

Fiona's Timeline

CHAPTER 7
FROM WOMB TO WORLD

'I'm trying to get Mummy... I can't get Mummy... Nanny won't wake up!'

The panicked words uttered by a three-year-old child!

That three-year-old child was my eldest daughter, Maya, who, having spent the morning alone with her nan, greeted her grandad with this news upon his return home. Tears streaming down her puffy pink face, she was desperate for her mummy. But her mummy wasn't there!

Instead of nursing my darling daughter through one of the biggest traumas of her life, I was in a coffee shop 23 miles away, nursing a smooth, comforting mug of hot chocolate, munching on a bacon roll and lapping up some much-needed 'me time'. I'd been visiting my parents and popped into Birmingham city centre for some solo shopping, revisiting that forgotten feeling of freedom. That was until the phone rang. Then the world that I had known fell apart in an instant! My mum was in an ambulance on her way to hospital, having been found unresponsive following a severe brain haemorrhage. The extent of the damage was so severe that she never regained consciousness.

Never in a million years would I have imagined that leaving my daughter to spend quality time with her grandmother could inflict such a shatteringly deep wound. What does that do to an innocent child who up until that point had been protected with a passion?

But Maya wasn't the only child affected. I was in fact pregnant. What about the 12-week-old foetus growing inside me?

Even at that age, she had already experienced trauma. It had been only five weeks earlier that my sister-in-law Jayne had died from cervical cancer. Little did I know then that her death was to be the first of many that we would suffer over the course of that pregnancy, and the opening scene for a further 10 years of suffering and loss.

CELLULAR MEMORY: INTRAUTERINE TRAUMA

So, as my second daughter, Lyla, was growing in the womb, she was exposed to a chemical cocktail of trauma as I was floored by one sudden death, then the next, and the next.

The impact of traumatic or stressful early life events, such as those experienced by Lyla, is something none of us expect to need to prepare for, but whilst so much trauma and loss during pregnancy may be unusual, my experience was nothing new. There have been women all over the country, all over the world and throughout time who have been unable to protect their baby from trauma, no matter how hard they tried.

Traumatic events alter the chemical set-up and internal environment during gestation and can therefore influence the physical development of the baby at whatever stage they have reached at the time.[1] This form of trauma is termed intrauterine trauma.

Cellular Memory

I remember my sheer terror and self-recrimination when consuming the research literature on intrauterine trauma, and how final those words felt to read. Science talks of cellular memory, also termed body memory, suggesting that memories and personality traits can be stored outside the brain and in the cells of the body. This idea, that non-brain tissue can store memory, is believed by many scientists to be an impossibility; however, anecdotal evidence from organ transplant patients such as those discussed by psychoneuroimmunologist Dr Paul Pearsall in his book *The Heart's Code*,[2] does call this into question. Research by cellular biologist Dr Bruce Lipton reaffirms this and shows that cellular memory can be transferred from a mother to her unborn child.[3]

During pregnancy, not only do the nutrients in the mother's blood nourish the foetus through the placenta but a whole host of hormones are released, alongside the chemical signals generated by the emotions she experiences. According to Lipton, chronic or repetitive negative emotions or trauma in the mother can biochemically alter the expression of the genes in the child.[4] These chemical signals have been found to activate specific receptor proteins in the mother's cells, as well as in the foetus, essentially pre-programming how the child will adapt to their environment and triggering physiological, metabolic and behavioural changes as a result.[5] We start to see, therefore, how a child who has experienced a stressful environment in the womb can become particularly susceptible to similarly stressful situations in the world, because they're effectively primed for a highly reactive fight-or-flight response and therefore also primed for illness and disease if this stress response remains activated.

Such findings are reaffirmed by the work of psychiatrist Thomas Verny, whose research confirms that when a pregnant woman's stress hormones travel through her bloodstream to the womb following acute or chronic stress or trauma, the same stressful response is activated in her unborn child.[6] Verny's studies also show that when under such extreme and constant stress in the womb, babies are more likely to be premature, lower in weight, hyperactive, irritable and colicky; some are even born with ulcers or thumbs sucked raw.[7,8]

There are also numerous studies documenting how a pregnant woman's stress, even as early as the first trimester, can affect her child. One such study[9] examined the relationship between pre-natal stress and the neurological development of the infant. The researchers measured the stress-regulating hormone cortisol in the amniotic fluid of 125 pregnant women and found that babies exposed to increased cortisol in the womb, as early as 17 weeks after conception, exhibited impaired cognitive development at 17 months old.

Now I recognize this can be a hard read for some of you, believe me! As someone who has inadvertently passed the impact of my own trauma on to my children, I know how hard it can be. But as a psychologist, I also know the value of the conscious awareness and acceptance of what you carry. Such knowledge can cultivate self-compassion, further self-understanding and facilitate healing for all involved. As with anything personal, you may have a deeply emotional response to the words on this page, which is perfectly natural, and I will say once again, please do seek external support if necessary.

Connecting with your response to this chapter can provide helpful insights to explore in your journalling. Do remember, however, that the meaning you then choose to associate with this knowledge is down to you, and please be exceptionally mindful of not turning this into self-blame. Show yourself some kindness and compassion, and consider that you can't control the outcome of every situation, but you can influence how you view it (and yourself).

If you're a parent who feels guilty for unintentionally causing harm to your child, recognize it was not in your power to prevent this. On the other hand, if you're a child who experienced an inhospitable environment in the womb (sadly, I can raise a hand here also), take solace from the fact that when you work through this on all the levels of the Self, from the position of parent or child, you can most certainly change the thoughts, feelings and energy surrounding it and emerge whole.

TRAUMA IN THE WORLD

For me, an additional trauma when pregnant with my second child was that I was utterly convinced I'd seen in my dreams that one of us was about to die!

Having repeatedly, and accurately, foretold numerous events throughout my whole life, I didn't know whether this was just a normal reaction to the accumulation of trauma and loss endured over the course of the pregnancy or a preview of the next catastrophe that was about to unfold. All I could do was wait. Only time would reveal the truth, so my main task at that point was to work on letting go of the fear and limiting any over-identification with that particular outcome. Instead, I put my energy into constructing an alternative ending where we would both survive, generating, positively reinforcing and feeding a future-Self timeline that stretched past the birth and all the way out into the distance.

We'll talk more of this concept later, but it is certainly something I would encourage you to have an awareness of, and not just in difficult times. Always pay attention to what future outcome you're constructing. Are your actions, beliefs and values in alignment with the future-Self you wish to become and the future life you wish to live? Be sure to energetically feed the outcomes you wish to grow and to starve the ones you don't. With the vibration of positive emotion and conscious thought, repeatedly visualize how such future events will play out in the positive – rewire *that* reality into your brain with *all* your senses. This shifts you out of the passivity of autopilot and can help to prevent the unconscious branching out of an unwanted reality.

But what of my own reality? The moment I'd feared my whole pregnancy was upon us, signified by a particular midwife coming on shift and standing at the foot of my bed. Her name badge was already emblazoned in my memory from the many times this scene had played out in my dreams. My body flooded with ice-cold terror the moment I caught sight of her name. *Everything* was playing out just as I'd foreseen it, which meant that the time had arrived for my baby or me to die!

It was also time to push, and push I did, but instead of cries of life, my efforts were met with deathly silence. My body limp, I had nothing left to give as the medical staff ushered me to release the rest of my baby's body into the world. I was spent. I just knew she was gone... and so was I! Submerged by my grief, I sank, despondent at every level of my being, feeling I had no choice but to resign myself to the horrors that lay ahead.

Moments later, however, Lyla's first cry signalled that we had in fact *both* made it through alive!

For a short time after the birth, we consumed the comfort that came with a ceasefire from the barrage of bereavement, yet in reality the war had only just begun. A mere nine weeks later, we were faced with the sudden and unexplained death of my 36-year-old brother, Mark.

Unaddressed Trauma

In situations like this, life dictates we move along with the new, fill up our cup with a big dose of gratitude and banish to the shadows all that no longer serves us. I had a healthy baby girl who needed me, so what was the point of focusing on anything else? I had no choice but to move on to the endless laundry, the sleepless nights and the cries of hunger.

But what of the turmoil that came before? What of the future that, for a time, however fleeting, became a reality – until a new reality came along? At that moment, at all levels of my being, I was giving birth to a baby girl who had already died, and in those few painful minutes a new future-Self was born that would bear that burden. That future may have been wiped from the slate, but a part of that moment would live on energetically.

Such trauma, whether acknowledged or not, remains forever present if left unaddressed and unexpressed. Just because the eventual outcome of a situation is far better than it could have been doesn't mean we should dismiss or minimize any of the wounds suffered along the way. In fact, the very act of leaving such trauma unattended enlists an energetic gatekeeper to ensure any conscious evidence of its occurrence remains locked away. Although this may enable a moving on, it soaks up the vital resources and life-force necessary for connecting fully with an enjoyment of the now.

Take my client 'Alice',* for example, a highly competent, professional lady in her late thirties struggling to navigate life with a pre-schooler and a six-year-old son. At least one of her sons, perhaps both, could meet the diagnostic criteria for dyslexia, attention deficit hyperactivity disorder (ADHD) and even autism. Accordingly, much of Alice's time as a mother had been beset by numerous challenges. Even her journey *into* motherhood had been extremely tough, including several failed embryo implantations and miscarriages, both prior to and during *nine* traumatic cycles of IVF treatment.

I began working with Alice when her eldest son was around eight months old. She was suffering from post-natal depression, insomnia and anxiety. With her unrelenting standards and near-constant negative rumination, she was struggling to feel connected to her son and feeling inadequate as a mother, dismissing and undermining her every maternal instinct through a fear of not obtaining the perfection she *so* expected of herself.

I'm introducing Alice to you as she, like Fiona and so many of my other clients, is a prime example of someone who has needed to mentally disconnect from the repeated trauma she has endured to 'just keep going' and function in the world. The demands of motherhood outweigh the demands for past trauma to be acknowledged and expressed. Not only that, but through some kind of survivor guilt, or loyalty to those hampered by less desirable outcomes, she deems anything less than an expression of gratitude for her current situation to be totally unacceptable and self-indulgent. During our work together, this has most notably shown up through a distinct lack of self-compassion and a dismissal of 'all that came before the miracle of being

---

* Names have been changed to maintain confidentiality.

blessed enough to complete my family'. Regardless of how tough life is now, it's met with the same responses: 'I should be grateful for what I have; many people have life much worse,' 'I'm the one that wanted children; many people never have them,' 'I should just stop complaining and get on with it.' It seems impossible for Alice to give herself permission to express her very real and understandable response to any difficulties in the now.

Sadly, we live in a world where toxic positivity has taken root and this denial of the whole experience of the Self is all too often reinforced by society. It's important therefore that we learn to be with, rather than to escape from, the parts of the Self touched by suffering. Should Alice be denied the right to acknowledge and express her exasperation when struggling with her children, just because she's grateful she finally has them or because she feels bad that others do not? By dismissing the reality of her experience and denying herself compassion, she is likely to be exacerbating her anxiety and insomnia and creating the perfect conditions for her former depression to thrive once more.

Being grateful that one hardship is over doesn't change how difficult the next one can be. Equally, the suffering of another need have no influence over how deeply we relate to our own. This may sound harsh if you're someone who thinks of others first, but really, one has no influence over the other. We can express gratitude for what we have *and* feel disappointed that it doesn't quite measure up to expectation; we can feel sad about someone else's circumstances *and* joyful about our own; and we can process our suffering *and* still get through daily life.

Are you starting to see how important it is to acknowledge, accept and process the difficult times you have encountered on your journey? We're quite rightly taught to show gratitude for what we have, and there is much research that attests to how this outlook improves our physical[10,11] and psychological[12,13] health, but it should never come at a cost to the integrity of the Self.

I wonder if you've done this in *your* life. It doesn't need to be anything really dramatic, or traumatic, but if a future reality has been constructed and elevated vibrationally due to a heightened emotion, then, like a sucker sprouting from the root of your timeline with no future to grow towards, there it remains – connected and feeding from the energetic field – frozen in time and stunted in growth!

ACKNOWLEDGING YOUR ADVERSITY

It might be useful now to take a moment to complete the Adverse Childhood Experiences (ACE) questionnaire,[14] which you can access on my site (*page xxvi*). This is a tool used to assess your exposure to potentially harmful childhood experiences. It was developed by the Centres for Disease Control and Prevention (CDC) and Kaiser Permanente to study the relationship between adverse childhood experiences, such as abuse, neglect and household dysfunction, and negative health outcomes later in life.[15]

The reason this study was so important was that it showed a strong correlation between adverse childhood experiences and a variety of health and social problems in adulthood. High scores on this questionnaire have been linked with chronic physical and mental health problems, substance abuse issues, financial problems, risky sexual behaviour, poor academic performance and even criminal behaviour. You can find more information about these outcomes on the Centres for Disease Control and Prevention website.[16]

Completing this questionnaire will not only bring more insight into what you are carrying from the past but also where you find yourself in the present. Once you have completed it, add to your timeline any additional experiences you might have missed or dismissed, along with any difficulties surrounding your birth that you're aware of. Be sure to consider not only the environment within the womb but also the environment outside it – any bereavement or trauma suffered by your parent or parents prior to your birth that could have impacted their attachment to you, along with any illness or marital difficulties they were facing, or even the responsibility of an older sibling in need of care.

Take a moment to gather this information and consider some of the journal prompts below for guidance.

Processing the Past

Your Birth Story

Journalling your time in the womb and your birth can be a valuable exercise if you are seeking to release pre-natal trauma. However, this can be a complex and potentially triggering process, so be sure to take care of yourself and seek support from a mental health professional if needed.

What do you know about your own birth story?

What was your mother's emotional and physical state during her pregnancy with you and during your early years? Was she under particular stress or subjected to trauma, illness, bereavement, health complications or any significant life events that might have impacted your experience or development in the womb or after?

How might this have shaped who you are today? Do any fears or anxieties come up when you think about this time? Do you have any physical, emotional or behavioural patterns or symptoms that may be connected to these experiences?

It's so important to make peace with these past experiences and release the associated energy that's locked into your nervous system before it manifests as illness in the body or plays out through the generations yet to come.

Inner Dialogue Work

When there are parts of you that need to be heard and healed, you can journal a dialogue between them and a 'wiser self'. If the wound occurred in childhood, conduct a dialogue between your childhood Self and your adult Self. If the wound occurred in adulthood, conduct a dialogue between your current Self and your future healed Self.

In this exercise you mentally reverse roles with yourself anywhere along your timeline, beginning as the hurt part and bringing in the wiser part to support and guide the vulnerable Self and encourage them to express what they couldn't at the time of the event.

Here's a dialogue Fiona might have with herself:

Child Self: I'm Fiona. I'm seven years old and have been told my mummy has died. It's my fault! I was always making her life difficult…

Adult Self: Hi, Fiona, it sounds like you're struggling with your mum's death. It's really hard to lose someone you love and often people blame themselves, especially when they can't find another reason for it. You say you feel you were always making her life difficult. What makes you believe that?

Continue the inner dialogue for as long as you need to. When it has run its course, end the conversation by writing a few sentences in closing, or perhaps write a letter to your child/distressed Self from where you are today, telling them what you *now* know that you didn't then. An example of this for Fiona might have her adult Self focus on bringing in some empathy and compassion for what she has been through, as based on how she relates to herself in the present, this is certainly something she never got the chance to internalize from her caregivers growing up. Children often carry shame and blame, so normalizing their response to events and ensuring they know they aren't responsible for what happened is of paramount importance for healing. The letter might also express gratitude towards her for carrying on despite her difficulties and how that has allowed her adult Self to develop certain strengths and qualities that have helped her to succeed in life.

Now, before we move on to improving your current situation and your future, we need to slip further back down that timeline towards any unnoticed distress signals from your ancestors that may have been silenced out of range – now is the time to hear them!

CHAPTER 8

AWAKENING YOUR ANCESTRY

Whether you have children or not, the content and exercises in these chapters are relevant to everyone. We all belong to a genetic line, we were all once children, we had parents, we had grandparents, so when considering the research, there is no escaping that the past does not start with your birth, and its impact does not stop with your death.

Assuming you have completed the Timeline of Transformation, you'll have already come face to face with some of the difficult encounters from your past that may be influencing your present. Deep down, some of you might even feel you're to blame somehow – that you're the source of all this turmoil.

What if there's evidence that the origins of these hardships may have nothing at all to do with you? What if they're not your fault at all? Could knowing that help you shred this sabotaging sheet of shame?

TRANSGENERATIONAL TRAUMA

What I have learnt through my life experience and clinical practice, then later confirmed through consulting the research literature, is that the roots of challenges may not reside in your immediate life circumstances, or in the events of your past; nor might they be the result of chemical imbalances within the brain or the gut. The origins of your stresses and strains may actually link back to the lives of your parents, your grandparents, even your great-grandparents. As such, the solutions to your suffering may be just as likely to lie within the stories of these relatives as within your own.

Who would have thought it? Whilst you may have grown up knowing you inherited your green eyes from your gran, your freckles from your father and your long legs from your mum, that very DNA may have also bestowed upon you a whole lot more. Like an echo from the distant past reverberating through your soul, trauma can be passed on via genes, as well as via dysfunctional thoughts and behaviours that have been constructed to deal with that trauma and then passed on thereafter.

Research in the fields of epigenetics (*epi* meaning 'above' genetics), cellular biology, neurobiology and developmental psychology reaffirms the importance of exploring this transgenerational trauma. Such findings emphasize how at least three generations of family history should be considered if we're to recognize the mechanisms behind repetitive patterns of trauma and suffering in the present.

Such second-hand traumas are like subconscious stowaways silently eating away at our wholeness, our resources and our potential. We must consider their impact in addition to any limitations or difficulties we were born into in terms of our family circumstances, for example abandonment, toxicity in our external environment, or situations generating repetitive stress, or that were deemed unsafe. We must purge our Self of these energetic parasites silently sapping us of the very life-force necessary for our health, our happiness and our healing.

If you used my template for the timeline, you might have noticed there were sections across the bottom designed to accommodate this insight and to facilitate an even deeper level of connection to these unacknowledged areas of your story: generational trauma, before/during birth, family circumstances. Significant complications in these areas, whether you know about them or not, have the potential to significantly impact your present and your future.

INDIVIDUAL RESILIENCE

When it comes to trauma, no two people are alike. The stress response is triggered by a *perceived* threat, and that perception will vary from person to person. So, you may find you're pretty resilient, bouncing back like a rubber ball every time tragedy is thrown your way. Your best friend, however, might be totally floored by the slightest whiff of a weighty word. We must always take into consideration the importance perception plays in our response to threat. It's for this reason that I proposed our definition of trauma should encapsulate any situation that has the capacity, for whatever reason, to activate and overwhelm our stress-response system, diminish our capacity to cope and trigger a disconnect from our authentic Self.

So, as well as possible intrauterine trauma, cultural trauma, developmental trauma, family dynamics and external environment, our timeline might also incorporate levels of resilience and desire to make a change. We can make that change. When we know the effects of our past, we can predict its impact on our future and choose to steer our life in a *new* direction – to a place of our choosing.

COLLECTIVE TRAUMA

The fallout from trauma isn't always obvious in the lived experience of all. I write these words knowing full well that as a white, educated, professional, British female, I'm the product of the level of privilege I carry, alongside the inequalities and traumas I've experienced personally and inherited from generations past.

There are, however, numerous cultures and populations who have been beset by bigotry and bias, living day to day drenched in discrimination and danger. Such oppression, whether current or past, can leave a stain that can be hard to transcend without a long-lasting change in society.

If we are to foster a framework for the future that is free from such prejudice, that too begins by looking back and becoming more aware of our own past-Self and all those influences that have shaped the person we have become in the present. The feelings, fears, behaviours and thoughts we've inadvertently adopted breathe life into a cycle of suffering that is passed on from one generation to the next, both individually and collectively. So, it's time now for us to travel back even further along our timeline, so we can connect with the potential impact from generations past!

Wherever in the world you and your family originated and whatever culture or society you were born into, there is no escaping that somewhere along that generational timeline, your ancestors, known and unknown, have been exposed to one form of trauma or another. Whether that wounding took place through disease, disaster, deprivation or degradation, according to the science, it may very well be living on through you.

Let's take a look at that science now.

THE SCIENCE

Epignetics

For years we've been taught that we're powerless to alter our biology. So, if breast cancer, cardiovascular disease or diabetes has been a component of your family DNA, there has been the assumption that this disease will soon come knocking on your door. However, the pioneering cell biologist Dr Bruce Lipton has demonstrated through his research that this isn't necessarily the case, due to his work in epigenetics.[1]

Epigenetics is a comparatively new science on the biological block and has shown that it's the signals from the *environment* that control the behaviour and physiology of our cells, including turning specific genes on or off.[2] This is certainly an area to watch, with other recent studies in areas such as cancer,[3,4] congenital heart disease[5] and even Alzheimer's, Huntington's and Parkinson's disease[6] suggesting epigenetics is a fundamental factor in both the development and treatment of inherited illness. This means we no longer need to buy into a belief system that limits us to experiencing the consequences of the genes we were born with – genes said to be responsible for 40 per cent of all illnesses.

To understand the importance of this, we will briefly review evidence from a significant number of studies that illustrates how the traumatic experiences of a parent can influence the gene expression and stress patterns of their children and future generations.

Epigenetic tags are the chemical signals in the cell that attach to the DNA and act like gatekeepers. They tell the cell to either activate or silence a specific gene, thus regulating gene expression and causing it to function in a specific way. Research has shown that epigenetic tags can account for differences in how we regulate stress later in life[7] along with whether subsequent generations gain a predisposition for physical or emotional health difficulties.[8,9]

Behavioural Biological Inheritance

Interestingly, it's not just physical traits, mental illness and diseases that are inherited from generations past. Over the many years I have been assessing and working with clients, I have often noticed patterns, challenges, behaviours and an outlook on life that were also present in previous generations of their family, in addition to abuse, addictions, challenges within relationships and family feuding, to name but a few. It often seemed as if my clients had somehow been pre-programmed by the experiences of their close relatives and thus strangely blind to all other possible realities.

Looking back to Fiona's timeline (*page 118*), you can see the repetition of familial patterns in the form of poor attachments, trauma, suicide, depression and loss.

The notion that behaviours can be passed down from one generation to the next could until recently only really be explained through learned behaviour and an adaptation to the inherent environmental conditions; however, this is now seen as taking place through biological mechanisms. It suggests that some behavioural traits may be inherited through genetics and others through epigenetic mechanisms in a process called transgenerational epigenetic inheritance.

Transgenerational Epigenetic Inheritance

We know that all the cells in our body contain the same set of genes, but they don't all look or behave in the same way. Epigenetics plays an important role in shaping the identity and function of cells, for example whether they become muscle, bone or skin during development. Contradicting the traditional view that inheritance occurs only through the DNA code that is passed down from parent to offspring, epigenetics helps us to understand that our genetic blueprint is just the starting point for our development, as influences from the environment can shape us emotionally, psychologically, behaviourally and biologically from as early as conception. This shaping process continues throughout our lives, constantly influencing our health and wellbeing.

On that basis, as we can change the conditions of our environment and also shift our perception, we clearly have the capacity to free ourselves from the lottery of genetic determinism and create the alternative conditions necessary to enhance our lives!

Inherited Trauma

An expert in the field of post-traumatic stress disorder (PTSD), Rachel Yehuda, PhD, a professor of psychiatry and neuroscience, has examined the neurobiology of PTSD in Holocaust survivors and their children, as well as in survivors of the 9/11 terrorist attacks. In doing so, she has provided considerable evidence that trauma can be passed down from one generation to the next.

When analyzing a particular region of a gene associated with stress regulation in adults who had experienced trauma during the Holocaust, she found the same epigenetic tags on the same part of the gene in both the parents *and* their subsequent children who had not experienced that trauma. After comparing the results with those of Jewish families living outside Europe during the war, Yehuda was able to confirm that the genetic changes in the children of Holocaust survivors were specifically related to the experiences of their parents.[10]

Her discoveries with this population mirrored her findings when assessing children born to women who were pregnant at the time of the World Trade Center attacks and subsequently developed PTSD. This research also revealed that children born to trauma survivors had low levels of the stress hormone cortisol, a finding also prevalent in their parents.[11] Such observations are extremely important, as although stress is most often associated with high cortisol levels, in chronic PTSD or when someone has been subjected to prolonged stress, the opposite can occur, as over time cortisol production can become dramatically impaired. If you remember, we can crash into a shutdown state after prolonged stress, so discovering cortisol suppression in the children was a significant indicator of epigenetic inheritance.

It's also important to note that when cortisol levels are compromised, so is our ability to regulate emotions, adapt to change and manage stress effectively. These characteristics were also evident in the children, and this is certainly something I have observed as a challenge for my daughter Lyla, and the numerous children I have worked with, also. Not only this, Yehuda also notes that several stress-related disorders, including PTSD, chronic pain syndrome and chronic fatigue syndrome (CFS), are associated with low blood levels of cortisol,[12] which again is certainly what I see with many of my clients and is illustrated by Fiona, who most definitely carried inherited and personal trauma and has recently received a diagnosis of fibromyalgia, which is effectively another name for CFS.

When considering all these research findings, I'm sure it's already becoming apparent to you that if you have such a biological and energetic inheritance due to parental or ancestral trauma, you'll already have little capacity in your stress bucket, despite not being directly involved. Genetic changes and impaired cortisol production may also mean you're potentially coming into the world pre-programmed for illness and disease, and are much more likely to experience difficulties with adapting to change, managing stress and regulating your emotions. There is even evidence that children of trauma survivors are three to four times more likely to struggle with depression and anxiety and engage in substance misuse when *either* parent has suffered from PTSD,[13] so that's something to consider also.

Reflecting on Your Inherited Trauma

How do these findings relate to you and your life?

Can you see any behavioural patterns or illnesses that might have been passed down through your family line?

Are there difficulties or issues you carry that just don't feel as if they belong to you? Perhaps they don't, or at least you may not be solely responsible. My hope is this research is just what you need to begin bringing in a little self-compassion – the first step towards healing.

Rachel Yehuda suggests these epigenetic changes are to biologically equip us to handle the traumas that our parents went through, thereby providing us with environmental resilience that allows us to effectively adapt to similar stressful situations that we may face.[14] This inherited adaptation becomes detrimental, however, when there is a mismatch between the epigenetics and the actual environment we are exposed to. So if someone remains in a state of high reactivity even when there is no danger in their environment, they could become predisposed to developing stress-related disorders and illnesses.[15]

Can you now see the importance in having an awareness of what occurred before and during your birth? You don't necessarily need to know the specifics, although if you're anything like me, you might *want* to 'know your story' on an intellectual level. Do remember, however, the thinking mind is only one of the many ways in which this information can be stored and processed, and we also have the communication of the body, the expressions of the heart and the language of the soul to help us shift and alchemize this energetic burden.

The past isn't the only place we can find such knowledge either; if unprocessed and impacting the Self, such events are playing out in the present moment, and therefore can be found and healed from there too. This can then radiate healing back down through our ancestral timeline in the quantum.

The most fundamental aspect of healing such trauma is knowing there is likely to be some there. We then get to know the energetic impact that carrying this has on our thoughts, our feelings, our behaviours and our relationships. Just acknowledging our ancestors' hardships and knowing the aftershocks may be living on through *our* timeline can be all we need to gain the awareness and self-compassion necessary to let go of this legacy and release our future-Self and future generations from its grasp.

Cellular Memory: Evidence of a Three-Generation Chain

Our shared history with our parents begins before conception. In our most primitive biological form as a non-fertilized egg, we already share a cellular environment with both our mother *and* our grandmother, as the precursor cell of our egg was present in our mother's ovaries when our grandmother was around five months pregnant. This is the same in the paternal line.[16] This means that at that time, all *three* generations were exposed to the same biological and energetic environment, thus what impacts one can impact all!

Research on the multi-generational effects of stress in humans is time-consuming, due to the length of time it takes for a new generation to emerge, so researchers have turned to studying mice. With a genetic similarity of 99 per cent to humans, it's reasonable to assume there will be a comparative outcome. These studies have shown that stress, including maternal separation, does in fact alter gene expression in mice for at least three generations, along with generating behavioural patterns characteristic of anxiety and depression.[17]

These findings were mirrored in experiments on rats. Again, the stress pattern was observed in multiple generations.[18]

These findings have led researchers to propose that children born to parents exposed to traumatic or stressful events would *also* be likely to pass this pattern down to multiple generations, but human research-based evidence is still needed to state that with *full* certainty.

Another intriguing study on mice revealed that even traumatic memories can be transmitted across generations via epigenetic changes in DNA.[19] The experiment conditioned one generation of mice to associate a cherry blossom-like scent with electric shocks, resulting in increased smell receptors associated with that scent so they could detect it at lower concentrations. They also developed enlarged brain areas devoted to those receptors. Researchers were also able to identify changes in the mice's sperm. Which may explain why the subsequent two generations also exhibited the same changes in the brain, fear response and sensitivity to the scent, despite never having experienced it before.

These studies also illustrate that a child's development and health can be profoundly influenced by the parents' thoughts, attitudes and behaviours.[20]

Although these studies may initially appear bleak, they offer hope for the future. As our understanding of epigenetics continues to expand, interventions designed to mitigate the transgenerational effects of trauma could become standard practice. Findings already suggest that thoughts, inner images and a daily practice of visualization and meditation can positively alter gene expression.[21, 22]

We already have many tools at our disposal to help alleviate the effects of trauma and silence the ghosts from generations past that are haunting us in the present.

Creating Your Own Genogram

A genogram is an important tool for Self-awareness and can help you make sense of how your past experiences and current life circumstances fit within the larger context of your family of origin. See the example on the next page, illustrating a few generational patterns noticeable in Fiona's maternal line.

At a glance, it's very clear to see that at each generational level there is a repetition of disconnected relationships, emotional deprivation, addictions, affairs, suicide, abuse and trauma. The impact of which is now carried by Fiona and her daughter.

Follow these steps to create your own:

1. Consciously gather as much information about your family that you feel might be relevant to your current situation: physical and mental health issues, relationship difficulties, deaths, suicides, births, traumatic events, for example.

2. Do the usual environmental preparation for connecting with your Self and your energy body so you're sitting in the power. Take your time to cultivate this.

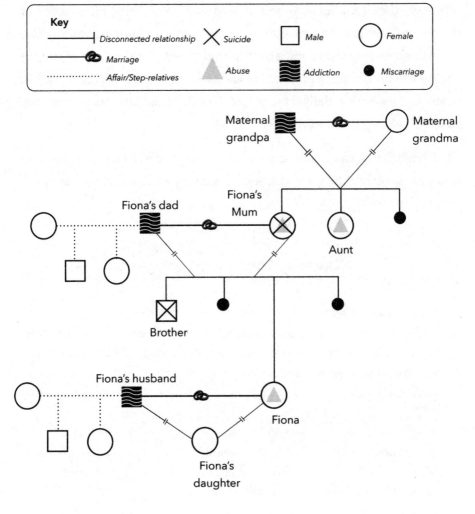

Fiona's Genogram

3. Think of your timeline as expanding out further than the number of birthdays you've had on this Earth and stretching back through the ancestral bloodline from which you emerged.

4. Set the intention that you're open to receiving as much guidance as necessary to gain healing for your own timeline and to those of generations past and yet to be birthed.

5. Begin drawing a genogram going back to at least the generation of your grandparents. If you don't know much about your family of origin, just work with what you do know. As I said earlier, this is just the intellectual element. The Release and Re-programming Method will work even without the detail.

6. Look for patterns and write down key themes and insights. Are there certain illnesses or conditions that seem to run in your family? Are there traumas or life events that seem to repeat? If family stories from generations back might relate to your life, for example slavery, war, famine, poverty and religious affiliations, then make a note of this too.

It's a sobering thought that where we are now is partially the result of the experiences of those who are long gone. Sleeping inside all of us are fragments of traumas that have perhaps been too great to find resolution in one generation and so the aftershocks have been felt through many generations and are creating fault-lines that can be felt forever more. More positively, processing and healing our own trauma will positively impact those who follow us. So, let's do this not just for ourselves, but for the generations yet to come.

CHAPTER 9

A LIFE BEFORE LIFE

Now, as The Psychic Psychologist, I can't possibly talk about the potential impact of what occurred prior to your birth without touching on past lives and reincarnation – the transfer of life-force, the soul or a consciousness stream into a new physical body following the biological death of the previous one.

Reincarnation has been a key feature of many cultures and religions for thousands of years and has large numbers of adherents all over the globe,[1] yet it remains a controversial topic.[2,3] What does the science say, and why is this of relevance to your healing and transformation?

From a purely materialistic perspective, it would seem impossible for people to remember past lives. However, if we once again consider the principles of quantum physics and the idea that consciousness underlies reality, with physical matter emerging from it, the concept becomes less far-fetched. If memories of past lives are stored in the non-physical realm of consciousness, rather than the physical brain or body, this could explain how some individuals are able to recall specific details of their previous lives. In addition, this theory could also explain how mediums and psychics access such information, as if downloading it from the iCloud of collective consciousness.

By taking quantum entanglement into consideration, where particles are connected across space and time, it's also plausible to suggest that information from past lives could be transmitted into the present via a quantum connection.

In the quantum, our existence isn't linear. I may talk of *past* lives and a timeline connecting our past, present and future Selves, but our lives don't necessarily stretch from birth to death. This is a three-dimensional perception of reality based on the lifespan of the physical body, but we exist on levels beyond this physical realm and can therefore transcend the limitations of time and space. From this perspective, it could be possible for our consciousness to move beyond the boundaries of a single physical body and through multiple incarnations or multiple dimensions of reality, where all the versions of ourselves exist simultaneously.

Quantum theory also provides a theoretical framework that could allow for the existence of parallel universes, with theories suggesting that each time a particle collapses into a single state, the Universe splits into countless versions of reality, each corresponding to a different outcome that could have occurred in a particular situation. This is currently impossible to test or prove through direct observation or experimentation, but, as in the film *Sliding Doors*, there could be versions of us in parallel universes living different lives based on having made different choices.

Yep, I totally get that this is hard to get your head around. As someone who has seen down timelines into other dimensions and witnessed alternate lives occurring in parallel to my own, I have a knowing of this reality based on my lived experience, but my brain still struggles to compute it all! However, the idea that our consciousness can simultaneously exist in multiple dimensions of reality and that our existence isn't limited to just one lifetime is part of many spiritual and metaphysical teachings and an area of active scientific research and speculation.

The survival of the soul, spirit or consciousness after physical death hasn't been scientifically proven, so it's understandable why many people discount it. However, we're not even able to observe the presence of consciousness in *living* physical beings, so how can we be expected to 'prove' its existence after death? Whilst there may be no scientifically verifiable methodology that can prove the existence of past or parallel lives, neither is there any scientifically verifiable methodology that can disprove it, so let's look at what we do know.

Following extensive scientific studies, psychiatrist Dr Ian Stevenson, former head of the Department of Psychiatry at the University of Virginia, believed the evidence was 'sufficient to permit a reasonable person to believe in reincarnation'.[4]

Dr Stevenson dedicated nearly 50 years of his life to the scientific investigation of this subject, finding evidence in support of accurate past-life recall from numerous children.[5] Having analyzed around 2,500 case files, both Dr Stevenson and his successor, Professor Jim Tucker, published numerous scholarly articles and books linking a patient's past-life memories to rare medical conditions and even birth defects, with nearly 20 per cent having scar-like birthmarks or deformities that closely matched the markings or injuries received at or near the death of the person whose life the child remembered.[6,7]

What's key for your journey is that in the research findings of both Dr Stevenson and Professor Tucker, behavioural and emotional difficulties consistent with these past-life identities were also present. For example, the children would often exhibit phobias in this lifetime that related to the death or negative experiences of the person whose life they remembered, and they would often display very strong emotional attachments to their supposed past-life families. The psychiatrists found a vast amount of detailed corroborated evidence in many of the case studies,[8] so much so that in a personal essay Dr Stevenson wrote: 'We all die of some affliction. What determines the nature of that affliction? I believe the search for the answer may lead us to think that the nature of our illnesses may derive at least in part from previous lives.'[9]

In his book *Many Lives, Many Masters*,[10] Dr Brian Weiss, also a psychiatrist, detailed the events that transformed *him* from sceptic to a firm believer in reincarnation. In it, he documents a series of therapeutic sessions with a patient called 'Catherine' who initially presented with panic attacks and anxiety. Having had no treatment success with traditional therapy, Dr Weiss then stumbled upon her past lives whilst using hypnosis. Past-life experiences that seemed to directly relate to her current problems were also noted, and when she had worked through them during regression therapy, her physical and emotional difficulties were said to greatly improve. The case of Catherine, and others, led Dr Weiss to conclude that past-life memories were rooted in actual experiences that had been carried forwards, rather than being simply products of a wild imagination.

Dr Weiss's work has been criticized by some, who state there has been a lack of scientific rigor. However, if the outcome of his work is to be believed, this, alongside the work of Dr Stevenson and Professor Tucker, points to the possibility of another way we might be affected by events from before this lifetime – in fact, from a different lifetime altogether.

As a hypno-psychotherapist myself, I have also been inadvertently taken into the realms of past lives with a number of clients, so I can attest to this process. What I can't confirm, however, is what's driving such memories. Having never objectively researched the details that clients recall, I can't confirm if they're a 'true' recollection of real-life events or whether the brain is simply using symbolism as a way to present information for emotional and mental processing. What I can say, however, is that having experienced such regression myself, during which I have 'visited' various lives, these recollections are in many ways more vivid and more emotionally charged than any memories from this one.

Interestingly, these lifetimes seem to mirror my own, as I *always* seem to be some form of healer, guide, medicine woman, tribal elder, witch or seer. Now, you might think my imagination might have conjured this up because of the work I do now, but connecting with these 'lives' occurred *before* I began working in this field, and back then this wasn't even on my radar.

The parallels don't end there. My death in many of those lifetimes involved drowning or suffocation (accidental and intentional), which corresponds to phobias I have repeatedly faced and re-experienced in this life and in dreams.

I have seen this with clients also. 'Anna'* comes to mind, as her improvement was nothing short of miraculous. She had experienced social anxiety and panic disorder since her late teens, to the extent that it prevented her from finishing university and getting a job. By the time she'd contacted me for help, her symptoms had progressed into agoraphobia and she hadn't been able to leave her home for seven months. Her world was getting smaller and smaller, yet within *one* month her symptoms had improved so much that she was out walking and enjoying meals with friends and family. We were using EMDR (Eye Movement Desensitization and Reprocessing), a trauma therapy, to help process the vulnerability she carried following her father's sudden death, when a 'rogue memory' popped in involving her last moments of life as a hungry and homeless teenage boy who'd been beaten and left to die. Despite her confusion, this memory felt as real to her as any other, so we treated it as such. Interestingly, her symptoms, triggered by the trauma of her father's death, had first emerged when she was a similar age to this boy, and they greatly and rapidly reduced once she had acknowledged his fear, vulnerability and abandonment.

As I write these words, I also remember a 'death memory' that surfaced spontaneously during my hypnotherapy training over 20 years ago. Previously, when walking through crowds of people, without warning, I'd

---

* Names have been changed to maintain confidentiality.

get bizarre intrusive, visceral experiences of someone stabbing me with a long blade through my stomach. The echo of terror and pain felt real, as if I had personally experienced such trauma. I could *even* feel the sense of satisfaction coming from my assailant. This connected 'memory' simply emerged spontaneously during my hypnotherapy training, and amazingly my harrowing experience in crowds has never occurred since. There was no therapeutic intervention; simply acknowledging this connection and impact within my body was enough to release it from my energetic timeline.

Make of this what you will – I'm simply presenting this information for you to explore and digest. My aim isn't to indoctrinate or influence you in any way, I simply wish to arm you with an awareness of what could prove to be helpful as you embark on your own journey to health and happiness.

The jury's still out for me. You may have noticed I tend not to jump into a binary narrative of true or false, good or bad – I'm comfortable with holding differing perspectives as possibilities all at the same time. As such, I'm able to suspend judgement and simply present my experience or knowledge. Whilst the evidence points to these experiences as being more than a creation of the mind, we can't truly know if we *actually* lived the life we remember or are tapping into an energetic imprint of that experience. I'm not even sure that it matters. The main point here is that it can often be a helpful process to release us from suffering.

So, whether you have a strange fear or phobia that can't be explained, keep re-experiencing the same relationship issues or health problems or just feel you've known someone before, perhaps consider that they *could* actually be unresolved lessons carried over from other lifetimes. This brings a fresh perspective into your life that could help you transcend your trauma, especially when you are stuck or re-experiencing the same situations again and again. In those instances, past lives could be worth exploring, but do so with a trained professional, as you can't necessarily predict what will surface, or know the emotional impact.

The key is always to lovingly acknowledge the lesson, release the energetic hold and gain closure, so you can use this knowledge to benefit your present- and future-Self. Through this process, you're able to gain genuine wisdom about how to make positive adjustments to your life.

Exploring Your Past Lives

For the reasons stated above it's not appropriate for me to teach you how to access your past lives here. Seek professional intervention for that. We can, however, gently open the doorway and allow your *inner*-tuition to guide you towards what might need healing.

1. First, note any connections you've made regarding past lives - situations, patterns, fears or emotional connections that just don't seem to align with your current life.

2. Place this alongside any themes from previous exercises and your timeline and genogram.

3. Now, let's gather more insight from your subconscious mind and request that it speaks to you through your dreams. Dreams can be very revealing when it comes to accessing details from past lives, especially recurring dreams and vivid dreams that make you question their reality. So:

   ~ Keep a journal by your bedside to capture any insights being communicated and notice any themes, particularly ones with a strong emotional charge.

   ~ Explore what might be playing out from this or another lifetime - are there unfamiliar places or people appearing repeatedly? Do you find yourself in a specific historical period?

   ~ Jot down anything significant, as you might then understand what your subconscious mind is trying to process or communicate.

The Garden of Remembrance

This is a more direct approach. Do this each night before you go to sleep:

1. Drop into the body and focus your awareness on your heart.

2. Placing your hands on your chest, imagine breathing in white light and it filling up and expanding out from the body.

3. Send out the intention to gain helpful insight and past-life information through your dreams.

4. Visualize a long hallway with doors either side and a large door at the end.

5. Walk down, open the large door and take seven steps down into your own *garden of remembrance*. Count the steps as you descend and take in all the sights, the sounds and the smells of this beautiful garden.

6. Walk over to a glistening stream – *the stream of consciousness*. Listening to the sound of the water and feeling the warm sun, look into the water. Allow yourself to rest and receive whatever information you need.

With repetition, your connection will strengthen, leading to deeper insight and recall. Information can come at any time – you could receive spontaneous downloads, gain insight upon waking, or maybe remember nothing at all. Keep a journal nearby to note down important revelations, but if nothing comes, just continue the process to enter a peaceful sleep, as you may gain conscious awareness later.

My advice is to begin each day free writing for around 10 minutes. Just write about your dreams or whatever else comes to mind, but do so before you do anything else (including picking up your phone). You'll be surprised how much more connected you become to your inner guidance – you just need to provide the time and space to let it flow.

Know also that even if you aren't aware of issues that relate to a life before life, you can assess and release the past through the exercises later in this book, so worry not, I've got you covered!

///

Now you've established an awareness of which events and situations from the past need healing, we'll move on to processing your painful past at each of the levels of the Self.

Remember, your past need not define your future, nor need it live on in the now. It may be playing out in the present, influencing your thoughts, your feelings, your actions and your energetic frequency, but you have the power to learn from those past experiences and to use that knowledge and awareness to facilitate healing and lasting change.

Let's do this!

CHAPTER 10

PROCESSING A PAINFUL PAST

Imagine your innate essence has become clouded by all the noise and static you've accumulated in your lifetime. As a result, you're no longer precisely attuned to the unique vibrational frequency that contains all your life potential. Instead of resonating as a multi-dimensional being, you're living in survival mode on the physical level, focused on fighting your illness, saving your relationship or buying your house, for example. It doesn't matter *what* specific events have occurred to shift that frequency dial to low; what matters is that there's interference, and that interference is detrimentally impacting your life, separating you from the full essence of your higher Self and thus preventing you from reaching your full potential. So, let me introduce to you my Hierarchy of Healing, which will enable you to do just that.

THE HIERARCHY OF HEALING

This is a healing protocol I have used to save myself and countless others from suffering. Now, you may have heard about Maslow's Hierarchy of Needs,[1] which states that an individual's most basic needs, such as safety, food, water and warmth, must be met before they can progress though to higher-level needs, such as having a loving relationship or achieving one's potential. In a similar vein, my Hierarchy of Healing has five levels of healing, as shown in the diagram below:

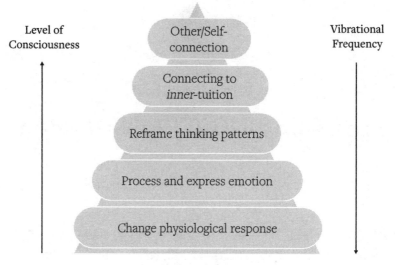

The Hierarchy of Healing

Just like Maslow, I propose that one level must be worked through so we can then heal at the next level. We must consecutively address each of these interconnected levels of the Self to fully eliminate whatever it is we wish to release from our lives.

I propose the disconnections and difficulties we face in life simultaneously impact us on all the levels and are expressed in the following ways:

- Unprocessed experiences – the physical level and in life experiences

- Unexpressed/suppressed energy – the level of emotion

- Harmful beliefs and maladaptive thoughts – the level of mind

- Denial/ignorance of our higher wisdom – the level of intuition

- Disconnection/abandonment in relationships – the level of Self-connection and other connection

Prioritize Physical Needs

If we remain in a place of suffering on a physical level, either through our body or within our environment, then it can be difficult to 'rise above' this, as we'll always be pulled down to the lowest level of difficulty. But by prioritizing our physical needs, such as self-care, nutrition, exercise, etc., whilst quietening the stress-response system and addressing any illness or impediment on the physical level of the Self, we can alleviate physical burdens that may otherwise hinder our emotional, mental and spiritual healing.

For example, you're going to struggle to connect with a fit and healthy future-Self if on a physiological level you're still eating junk food and not addressing your bad back, so are always restricted and in pain. Any attempt at shifting thoughts and emotions towards the future-Self will be shallow and short-lived because if you're not identifying as something new in the physical realm, then you're still rooted in that same old programming, and it's from there that the other levels grow.

Process and Express Emotions

Just as your physical state can keep you tied to your past conditioning, your emotional state can colour your perception and interpretation of events, which in turn shape your thoughts. If not expressed, these emotions, and the biochemistry they produce, can solidify into tangible discomfort, pain or illness in the body as they call to be attended to. By addressing and healing your emotions next, you in turn heal emotional bocks at the physical level, whilst also creating a healthier emotional landscape that positively influences your thoughts. Emotions reside in the body, so by addressing emotions before thoughts, you reduce energetic tensions and prioritize the release and healing of emotional burdens, creating space to challenge and reframe negative thought patterns so more positive and empowering thoughts can emerge.

Reframe Thinking Patterns

Through working with your thoughts next you can cultivate a mental clarity by challenging any limiting beliefs or ingrained thought patterns that may hinder your healing. Shifting from the vibrationally heavier thought streams can help you to maintain the developments that have occurred within the lower levels of the Self. Clearing any mental noise or negative thought patterns also allows you to connect with your values and purpose, so you can become more receptive to spiritual exploration and growth by fostering a more connected, open, and expansive mindset.

Connect with *Inner*-Tuition

Spiritual healing often involves transcending the limitations of the mind, so it's important to establish a certain level of alignment between your thoughts and spiritual aspirations, as it's through your thoughts that you send out your intention into the world. Aligning your thoughts with your spiritual values and intentions can facilitate a more integrated and harmonious spiritual journey and enables you to connect with your higher Self and your *inner*-tuition.

Make Other/Self-Connections

We can't be present to connect with another person if we remain disconnected from our Self, which is why relational healing comes last in the hierarchy. Healing the Self allows us to cultivate a deeper understanding of our own needs, values and boundaries, which is essential for fostering authentic and healthy connections with others. When we have a stronger sense of Self and have worked through personal healing, we're better equipped to engage in meaningful relationships based on mutual respect, empathy and genuine connection.

See the table opposite for how we address each level:

Physical Healing	Listening to the language of the body to connect in with your life lessons. Through addressing physical ailments and imbalances within the body, like chronic pain, illness or injury. In addition to traditional medicine, it may involve meditation, visualization, exercise, dietary changes, professional help, alternative healers and other lifestyle changes shown to improve overall physical health and wellbeing.
Emotional Healing	Addressing emotional wounds, traumas and limiting beliefs that may be holding you back from living authentically. This may involve therapy, journalling, energy work, mindfulness, meditation, movement, sound healing, emotionally expressive or creative outlets, music and other forms of self-reflection and introspection.
Mental Healing	Addressing negative thought patterns, limiting beliefs and self-sabotaging behaviours that may hinder your ability to connect with others and live authentically. This may involve cognitive behavioural therapy, journalling, cognitive restructuring, worry time, thought stopping, problem-solving, personal development, mindfulness practices or other forms of mental and emotional self-care.
Spiritual Healing	Connecting with your sense of purpose, values and spirituality. This may involve exploring different spiritual practices, connecting with nature, meditation, prayer, balancing your chakras, channelling healing, regularly connecting with your higher Self, developing your intuition and engaging in activities that bring a sense of awe, meaning and purpose into your life.
Relational Healing	Learning how to connect with others (and yourself) in a healthy, authentic way. Developing communication skills, active listening, deeper awareness of Self, attending to your own needs, setting healthy boundaries, cultivating empathy and compassion for Self and others. This connection must be present within the Self before it's possible to fully connect with another.

This Hierarchy of Healing protocol works for releasing anything from our life, not just illness. *Everything* affects us on all these levels – having a physical component, an emotional element and particular thoughts associated with it, which all impact our energetic frequency and how connected we feel to all that is within us and beyond us, spiritually or relationally. Not only are we impacted by events, people and illnesses on all these levels of the Self, for example, but our *inner*-tuition speaks its wisdom through the language of these levels also. So if we're disconnected from, don't understand or aren't even aware of this language, it will speak through our life circumstances until we have no choice but to take heed.

This is why you were encouraged to complete the quiz in the first chapter, to help establish how disconnected you've become from the Self on each of these levels. Remember, your results may have indicated you're disconnected in one particular area, but that also means you're most likely to be over-identifying elsewhere. The key here is to promote balance and healing through *all* the levels of the Self, so be sure to take the time needed to learn the tools that can be used for *all* the levels, rather than skipping forwards to just focus on one.

We start in this chapter with healing the dense, lower frequency energy of the physical body, as this serves as the foundation of our wellbeing.

OUR BODY SPEAKS OUR TRUTH

There are many reasons why we become disconnected from or overly preoccupied by the physical, leading to an imbalance within the body. I know for much of *my* life my energy and focus were placed on developing my thinking mind, and anything within the physical was dismissed or denied. For me, and a great number of people I have worked with, inevitable life circumstances then repeatedly present a way to reconnect and attend to the body's needs – most often through the onset of physical illness. When we're not present or not listening to the needs of the physical level, our body will speak our truth, in the only language it knows, until we take heed!

Have *you* ever stopped to wonder what the body might be trying to communicate to you about your past and current lifestyle? What unexpressed emotions or lessons have been missed as you've been living on autopilot, disconnected and disassociated from the physicality of your life? Perhaps there are things you've been saying 'Yes' to when the body has been quietly saying 'No'.

By taking the time to connect with our body and listen to its language, we may gain the valuable insight and wisdom needed to release ourselves from that story and make the positive changes necessary to live a more fulfilling life.

So, after all you've learnt so far, are you ready to listen? Are you ready to allow the body to become your teacher? To connect back with that physical imprint from the past and to finally allow it a voice? Well, that's exactly what we're going to do now.

I shall begin with an example of what you might find at this level of the Self. Here's what I've learnt through connecting with some of my own physical illnesses/symptoms (*see next page*).

Believe it or not, these are just a few of the physical manifestations of my life journey, but perhaps you can see how each physical symptom mirrors an aspect of some of the experiences I have shared with you earlier in the book.

I wonder if you might have found some significant events from your own life speaking through the body. I see this so often with my clients. My ex-husband, for instance, went permanently deaf in one ear once he was confronted by the impact of his infidelity. He did not want to hear or take in what I had to say, so much so that his body cut off his hearing that very same day – now that is surely no coincidence.

Physcial Ailment	Expression	Lesson
M.E./ Fibromyalgia	Physical expression of pain relating to unexpressed emotional pain that was not processed or released following the deaths. Intense fatigue due to low life-force. No desire to live, so ended up in a dark room unable to participate in life. Had nothing left for myself after being strong for others and helping everyone else!	Must nurture yourself to ensure a balance between what you're giving out and getting back. Express and process the painful emotions that have been suppressed. Senses are overstimulated with so much going on – break it down to reduce over-whelm. Nurture and increase self-care. Ask for help!
Mitochondrial Disorder	Empty energetic battery, with nothing left to replenish it, meant that I blocked the process of turning oxygen into life-giving energy. My body was literally expressing my disconnection with life.	Take space and time to regenerate and reconnect with life. Allow your batteries to replenish. Pace yourself. Find your reason for being here – your purpose. Allow and accept love. Work on gratitude. Live!
Inflammatory Bowel Disease	Too much toxicity and trauma to digest, so ended up eating painful emotions, unexpressed trauma, anger and grief, and causing an inflamed and ulcerated gut. I couldn't take up nutrients or anything else that's good about life.	Communicating more to process your trauma, but this time with an acknowledgement of unexpressed anger. Start to bring in the good (healing foods, energies, actions) to nurture the Self and bring in calm.
Legs suddenly buckling and giving way whilst walking	Physical manifestation of being unable to carry any more after too much pain and trauma in my life and taking on the emotional burden for others – life was just too heavy! Unpredictable onset of buckling felt like a replay of how the whole world was taken away from under me, with one trauma after the next, causing it to feel like there was no secure ground left in my life.	Do trauma work to process the past and work to release this on a somatic level too. Gain support from outside of yourself. Sometimes you need some scaffolding to hold you up when your world is crumbling. You need to accept that this is okay. Reframe your situation – you survived! Come back to the now!
Random Anaphylaxis to previously 'safe' food items	Physical manifestation of how unsafe life had become. Unable to take in anything good. The sudden and life-threatening nature of this mirrored how dangerous the world felt and, once again, was a replay of the sudden onset of the traumas in the past.	A reminder that life can be danger-ous and unpredictable – but you can survive! What was safe at any point may be taken away. Work through the trauma, and find safety and ground-ing in yourself through processing the past and releasing somatically. Trust!
Pituitary tumours	Fearing and blocking the spiritual aspects of life and living in a toxic internal and external environment.	Time to release the fear and recon-nect on all levels of the Self. Listen to your intuition.

It's not just our body that speaks our truth, those lessons speak through our life circumstances and our relationships too. Take my client 'Richard',* for example, eaten up by anger and grief over his brother's sudden death through alleged medical negligence, he never managed to express his inner turmoil. His thoughts, behaviours and feelings were focused on the bitterness he felt towards the National Health Service, whom he was fighting to hold accountable. His body soon reflected the repercussions of this war and his resistance to accepting this external reality, which saw his emotional suppression morph into a new battle in the form of terminal lung cancer.

Dr Gabor Maté, in his book *When the Body Says No,*[2] repeatedly talks of how the inefficient processing of emotions predisposes us to many illnesses, including cancer, with research by others also backing the suppression of anger specifically as being a significant factor.[3]

I present Richard to you here because his journey with me began at the exact same time I was consumed by thoughts of investigating my own brother's death. Richard's story mirrored my own, as I too believed my brother, Mark, had died a needless death prompted by medical negligence whilst in hospital. Faced with witnessing Richard's battle unfold before me, and seeing the heavy price he paid, enabled me to reflect on my own situation and the need to find justice for Mark. It felt as if another lesson was speaking to me through my physical reality, and that was that I should just let it go.

I'm hoping that even if you haven't experienced such events or illnesses yourself, by connecting with my experience, you'll see how important it is to listen to that *inner*-tuition, which comes in many forms. It's even played out for all to see in the words we choose. Those casual expressions we use all the time are revealing. I hear this often in the language used by my clients as they communicate to me the wisdom of the body that's beyond their

---

* Names have been changed to maintain confidentiality.

conscious awareness. Like my client 'Jane',* who said she was 'sick to the stomach' to think of how badly she'd been treated by her mother as a child. She was literally sick to her stomach, as her personal history was being expressed through the bulimia she'd endured since her teenage years. Mirroring her life experience, she couldn't take in any form of nurturing, even from herself, and held steadfast the control and high boundaries that had eluded her childhood. All this, along with severe IBS and anxiety, reflected the toxicity she'd had to swallow as a child, and the bulimia, a subconscious attempt to purge herself of the anger, trauma and grief that had been suppressed as a result.

And my client 'Sarah',† who was preoccupied by intrusive thoughts that she might go blind. This wasn't her main reason for seeing me and there was nothing wrong with her eyes, but I suspected that subconsciously she knew her son was stealing from her to fund his drug addiction but couldn't allow herself to see it! Interestingly, seven months later she missed a session as she was recovering from a medical emergency. You guessed it, it involved her eyes! One of her retinas had suddenly detached and she temporarily lost her sight.

'It just knocked me off-balance' is another very common phrase I hear, and almost exclusively from clients who have experienced a sudden trauma resulting in ear and balance issues.

Now remember, these interpretations are specific to each person's particular life story and life lessons. A stomachache for you will be likely to have a very different origin and meaning to a stomachache for someone else, and may need a different treatment approach. We may use the protocol as directed by the Hierarchy of Healing, but apply different tools at different levels. So, while physical symptoms may present in the same way, we have an individualized

---

* Names have been changed to maintain confidentiality.

† Names have been changed to maintain confidentiality.

and tailored approach to healing, including collaboration with our intuition for guidance.

I'm by no means asserting that we're 'causing' our own illnesses, nor would I ever suggest using this healing protocol as an alternative to traditional medical treatments and diagnoses. But we can have a huge impact in the healing of our own lives, of which illness is just one element. To do so, we must also connect with the wisdom of what's being expressed through our body so we can help generate the right conditions for health. We are the experts on ourselves, and it's through our body that we hold our unprocessed experiences and emotions. We just need to know how to listen, and where to look for those nuggets of wisdom waiting to be found.

This doesn't necessarily need to be what we're consciously carrying in our body right now; there might still be insight we need to connect with. For example, I no longer suffer from endometriosis; I healed this alongside my pituitary tumour at the age of 22. Now, I believe this was the body putting in place a boundary of safety that I hadn't provided for myself. I believe the origins of this went back to when I was 15 years old and became friends with a hotel entertainer eight years my senior. He was a resident dancer and fooled my parents into believing I was safe with him. They didn't seem to think I was vulnerable, and so, despite my inner voice, I told myself I was safe too – that was, until I wasn't! To this day, I don't fully know what happened on my last night of that holiday – he'd seen to it that I was intoxicated with alcohol, perhaps even drugged. But what I do know is that seeing his name and face on a double-page spread in a national newspaper a few years later – a 'wanted paedophile' who had escaped from prison and fled the country – was the beginning of acknowledging the parts of myself I had denied and hidden away. The reason I could heal the endometriosis, have children and remain healed was that I listened to my body. It was because I accepted and acknowledged the lesson, reclaimed my rejected femininity and never shut down my gut again. If, on the other hand, I'd continued to live in denial and suppressed this '*truth*', then in one way or another, it's likely the body would still be communicating this even now.

That's exactly what happened with my pituitary tumour – I neglected to continue with what had helped me to heal. Yes, I worked on the physical level, I released it on a mental level and I even processed the related emotions, but not only did I quickly disconnect from my spiritual Self once more, I remained in a toxic environment, both internally and externally, which is why 10 years later I found myself needing to heal myself again, but this time from not one but *two* pituitary tumours.

It can even be that we understand what's beneath our difficulties at a physical level but are still not ready to heal. My anaphylaxis still resurfaces at times, as I haven't fully managed to feel safe in the world. I behave as if food is dangerous and so it still is dangerous to me. Despite knowing I can heal from this, as shown though the research presented on dissociative identity disorder (DID) earlier, I still have some work to do to fully release my trauma, which is why it's still a part of my identity and still plays out in the now. We can see why when looking at the table opposite.

These examples illustrate that this work isn't a one-time-only fix, nor is it a miraculous healing that occurs simply with insight – it's a lifestyle of balance that needs to be maintained, a key part of which comes from having a clear connection with all the levels of the Self so we can listen to our *inner*-tuition and adapt accordingly!

Armed with all this, it's now time for you to look at what you're still carrying in the body from the past. Take the information you've just gained from the wisdom of the body, and alongside this, gather up your quiz results, your timeline, your genogram and all the knowledge gained relating to your past, and map out how this relates to how your life is being expressed in the now. Do this in whatever way works for you. Perhaps create some tables like mine, or do a new timeline specifically for illness/physical lessons, or generate a chart or diagram. When doing so, think through the following:

Physical Healing	I am still avoiding certain foods and acting as if they are dangerous to me. Due to the memory of previous physical experiences in the body due to anaphylaxis, I am hypervigilant and notice any change in sensation, effectively just waiting for it to happen again – we get what we look for.
Emotional Healing	I still have quite a bit of fear around foods and very likely still have many unprocessed emotions in my body relating to a lack of safety in the world. One of my symptoms is my throat closing up and simultaneous projectile vomiting. This is due to me blocking the expression of a tsunami of emotions and grief.
Mental Healing	I am still identifying as someone that gets random anaphylaxis to previously safe food items, so my thoughts and beliefs are in alignment with this. I believe it could happen again due to my past experiences and so am on high alert, fuelling the situation further.
Spiritual Healing	I've not listened/fully worked through the sudden barrage of trauma that continues to be replayed. The life-or-death feeling I experience during anaphylaxis episodes is exactly the same as the one I experience when I play out memories from the past, along with the sense that I am abandoned and alone in a scary world that can change at a moment's notice.
Relational Healing	I abandon my Self by not fully working through the root cause and project my fears onto others by subconsciously replaying the situation through anaphylaxis. They can then reaffirm the danger as I replay the trauma of feeling abandoned and having no one there to help, which is re-experienced in that moment when my face burns up and my throat starts to close.

Awareness

- What symptoms and illnesses do I carry/have I carried in my life? When did they begin and what was occurring in the months/years leading up to it?

- How is this being expressed in my body and what could it be a metaphor for?

- What unexpressed experiences from my life might be being expressed through my body?

- What lessons is my body trying to teach me or bring to my attention, and what do I need to attend to in order to recover/improve?

- What would I be *doing* differently if this wasn't present in my life?

Blocks

- What does my body need me to acknowledge and release physically so that I can begin to heal?

- What *stories* or life patterns do I need to resolve at this level of the Self to be free of this?

- What does all this bring into my life? What would I lose if I were to let it go? What's getting in the way?

- Who will I be without this in my life? Who do I need to become?

Make this specifically about the body and your behaviour, and be sure to correlate your physical ailments with your life events. I'm encouraging you to connect with your inner guidance for this, just like I did, but if you need some external suggestions in relation to a metaphysical interpretation of any physical ailments, then you could refer to books such as *Metaphysical Anatomy* by Evette Rose[4] or *Your Body Speaks Your Mind* by Deb Shapiro[5] for further guidance. I must stress, however, that it's advisable to go with whatever feels right to you and to generate your own interpretation based on your life circumstances, rather than blindly taking something suggested by someone else.

Once you've gathered the information you need, you can then use it to direct the work on the other levels of the Self.

For now, take a moment to connect with the body and feel into the main issue for you. If there's more than one, be sure to only work on one at a time. You might be surprised by the impact it has on the others, as they could very well be linked. Remember the toolbox of resources we've gathered together through the book – the safe space exercise, the container, breathwork, sitting in the power, etc. They will all help you to connect with your difficulties and regulate your emotions as you do so.

Connecting with the Body

Take a moment for reflection now, so you can connect with your physical body with those questions still in mind:

1. Begin with a body scan (*page 44*). What do you notice? Aches, pains, symptoms of illness?

2. Visualize a ball of white energy above your head, filling the body with each breath. Let it flow down through your central core and out through your feet, reaching deep into the Earth. Feeling grounded and connected, draw up this healing white light frequency from within the Earth.

3. Place your hands and awareness on your heart and connect with the wisdom and intelligence of your heart consciousness. Remain present in the body and set the intention to safely receive wisdom from the physical level across all space and time.

4. Write a letter to the body from the heart, expressing gratitude for its resilience and strength. Acknowledge any pain or challenges, past or present, and reflect on the lessons learnt from this chapter.

Express gratitude, compassion and understanding, and reflect on the emotions and thoughts that arise as you write.

5. Imagine the body's response to your letter. Listen to and journal on any messages, sensations or emotions that arise. Allow the body to express itself through your writing without judgement.

6. Switch roles or simply read your letter and the body's response aloud, allowing yourself to fully absorb the words and emotions expressed.

Close this exercise with a commitment to nurture and care for the body moving forwards. Resources that focus on processing the impact of trauma through the body, such as *The Body Keeps the Score* by Bessel van der Kolk[6] and *Waking the Tiger* by Peter Levine,[7] might prove helpful.

///

Assuming you stayed present and connected, you now have an awareness of what you are carrying in your physical body and insight into its origins. Let's now shift our focus to the level of emotion.

CHAPTER 11

CLEARING UNPROCESSED EMOTIONS

Emotions are complex psychological experiences that affect our physical and mental states, as well as our behaviour and actions. When we experience an emotion, it triggers the release of specific chemicals in the brain and body, including peptides. Peptides are biochemical messengers that act as signals to different parts of the body, including the nervous and immune systems. Neuroscientist Dr Candace Pert was the first scientist to establish this 'bodymind' connection through her work looking for the opiate receptor in the brain. In doing so she produced evidence that the body and brain are not separate. Her research, detailed in her book *Molecules of Emotion*,[1] indicated that repressed emotions and memories may be stored in receptors throughout the body, travelling in both directions, from the brain down into the body, and from the body up into the brain. This means that we can access emotional memory anywhere in that peptide/receptor network of the 'bodymind' and it may very well explain how body therapies based on massage and therapeutic touch can release stored emotional experiences and trigger profound transformation.

We're going to utilize a therapeutic technique called Emotional Freedom Technique (EFT) to help you process and re-programme what you are carrying from the past. But first, we need to identify and acknowledge what emotions are present.

AWARENESS AT THE ENERGETIC LEVEL OF EMOTION

Studies show that naming feelings can help with emotional regulation by diminishing the activation of the amygdala and other limbic regions.[2] This then has a knock-on effect, as it reduces the likelihood of a further physiological response such as a surge in adrenaline or cortisol, thus preventing increased blood pressure and heart rate. We often shy away from expressing how we feel, but simply putting words to it, for example stating, 'I'm feeling anger right now,' can help to release it and prevent the activation of the stress-response system, and thus any problematic behaviours or illnesses that could follow. The same is true if you're working with feelings stored from the past – these need validating and verbalizing too.

As we have already established, I'm proposing that each of our experiences is felt on all the levels of the Self; therefore, our emotions are as much a part of our body as they are of our brain. If you ask yourself how you know you're having an emotion, such as anger or sadness, it's often because you can feel it in the body as *feelings*. There is a physical experience in the form of sensations that are accompanied by specific biochemistry that influences us at an emotional level. There is also a specific energetic experience that comes along with that – I'm sure you can agree that the energetic feeling tone when you're down, depressed and lethargic is very different from the energy generated when you're feeling free, liberated and joyful. This is also true of thoughts that are generated. These will have a specific quality that corresponds with the emotion and energy generated by that physical experience too.

The idea of emotions having a different energetic expression in the body is supported by research that looked at the impact on the body of 14 different emotions.[3] Each of the 700 participants had to indicate where they felt different emotions in their body. The results were surprisingly consistent, even across cultures, which means we can potentially state that on average this is how people experience these emotions in the body. As a rule, happiness presents itself all over the body, from head to toe, while contempt is felt in the head and anger in the arms, fists, upper torso and head. This patterning could also relate to how such emotions can impact particular areas of the body, with certain emotions consistently generating particular physical illnesses and disease.[4,5] Such findings bring to light how such unexpressed emotional energy has the potential to become stagnant, excessive or out of balance, in line with Eastern philosophies that show how blockages in certain meridians cause illness in specific organs.

During a training exercise with Gordon Smith, it became apparent how emotional shifts affect the energy body too. Partnering up, one person sat and connected with a past memory whilst the other stood behind them, placing their hands above their shoulders to feel changes in their energy field. Interestingly, the energy field expanded and felt lighter with happy memories and contracted and felt heavy with traumatic or sad memories. This tangible experience showcased the influence our thoughts and emotions have on our energy field, potentially impacting our physical body and the people around us. Once you're comfortable with sensing your energy body and those of others, why not give this exercise a try and experience it for yourself?

Before we move on, let's look at the work of Dr David Hawkins, PhD, who developed a 'Map of Consciousness'[6] that outlines a scale of human consciousness and is based on his extensive research and clinical observations in the fields of psychiatry and spirituality. This hierarchical scale ranges from lower, denser emotions like shame, guilt, fear and anger to higher, more expansive emotions like courage, acceptance, love, joy and enlightenment. The model suggests that higher levels of consciousness have a positive impact on our wellbeing, relationships and overall life experience. By consciously choosing thoughts, emotions and actions that align with higher levels of consciousness, we can enhance our personal growth and spiritual development and contribute to the wellbeing of humanity as a whole.

All these factors point to why it's of paramount importance to release negative past experiences and unexpressed emotions from all the levels of the Self if we're to truly heal and transform our lives. When we're fully connected to the Self, we're aware of our emotions and express them in a way that prevents them from being suppressed and stored in the energetic or physical body.

Beginning to notice physical sensations in the body can help you to identify feelings, especially if you typically have trouble doing so, which is why it's important to regularly connect with the body through mindfulness practices, meditation and body scans.

Emotions can be disturbing, but we need to *feel to heal*, so staying present with disturbing emotions and becoming aware of their impact on all the levels of the Self can help them naturally resolve. This can also help us to figure out our triggers and learn more about our values and boundaries, so we don't need to feel that way moving forwards.

HOW TO HANDLE YOUR EMOTIONS

1. Acknowledge you're having an emotion.

2. Remain present without trying to change it.

3. Label the emotion if you can, using the identification table coming up.

4. Recognize the physical sensations, e.g., tension in hands, holding breath, trembling, etc.

5. Notice the thoughts present with the emotion and write them down for processing in the next chapter.

6. Once you have been present with the emotion, you can then use a coping skill if needed, e.g., breathwork or safe space visualization or

a tool to process it, for example Emotional Freedom Technique (EFT) (*page 187*).

In the table on the next page there are the eight core emotions as suggested by psychologist Robert Plutchik,[7] along with some associated feelings and possible physical sensations. This can help you to identify your emotions and make a connection between the emotional areas of the brain and the more conscious, logical areas.

It's from these core emotions that others are produced. For example, anticipation plus joy might form optimism, whilst anger and sadness might describe disappointment. Please be aware that at times a particular emotion may serve as a defence mechanism against another. This is particularly true if you were raised to suppress feelings that were deemed to be unacceptable, for example, 'Big boys don't cry.' This is indicative of a society that often encourages boys to express anger rather than sadness, which is why I so often see aggression and anger as symptoms of depression in men. Equally, many children are told not to be so emotional or sensitive, which can create a negative perception of expressing certain emotions. This can lead to the suppression of these emotions and generate feelings of shame or embarrassment when expressing them. For these reasons, it's crucial to be aware of the stories and programming that have shaped your emotional expression or suppression. This helps you identify your habitual patterns and explore emotions you may have dismissed or denied. Ask yourself:

- What attitudes relating to emotional expression was I exposed to as a child? What sayings did I hear? What did I learn?

- What have I been conditioned to believe about expressing emotions in general, and in relation to particular emotions – what's acceptable, what's not? What beliefs do I still carry now?

- What emotions *never* come up for me?

Emotions	Feelings	Physical Signs
Fear	Anxiety, apprehension, dread, terror, panic, powerless/helpless, frightened, scared, worried	Rapid heart rate, trembling, rapid breathing, stomach discomfort, diarrhoea, nausea, fight, flight, freeze, sweating
Anger	Irritation, resentment, frustration, annoyed, grumpy, hostile, mad, impatient, restless, cheated, vengeful	Clenched fists/jaw, tense muscles, flushed skin, rapid breathing, increased heart rate, increased blood pressure, sweating, tears
Sadness	Sorrow, despair, longing, isolation, loneliness, empty, melancholy, grief, regret, disappointment, hopelessness, helplessness, apathy, depressed	Crying, slumped posture, fatigue, loss of appetite, sleep disturbance, oversleeping, insomnia, slowed movement, muscle tension, physical heaviness, sighing, lack of motivation/ life interest
Joy	Happiness, excitement, elation, gratitude, bliss, love, optimism, awe, fulfilment, serenity, delight, wonder, glee	Laughter, smiling, increased vitality, bright eyes, warmth, playfulness, relaxed muscles and posture, glowing complexion, energy
Surprise	Disbelief, bewilderment, amusement, shock, curiosity, confusion, astonishment, intrigue, startled, thrilled	Raised eyebrows, wide eyes, dropped jaw, gasping, goosebumps, holding breath, startle response, dilated pupils, elevated posture, increased energy
Anticipation	Excitement, hope, optimism, eagerness, restlessness, tension, nervousness, apprehensive, impatience, intrigue, expectancy, trepidation	Butterflies in stomach, sweating, increased breathing rate, heightened focus, heightened sensory awareness, racing thoughts, body heat, restlessness, fidgeting, alert, attentive
Trust	Security, comfort, reliability, openness, peace of mind, safety, belonging, positive expectations, connection, closeness	Relaxation, calmness, warmth, relaxed muscles, soft facial expression, open posture, lightness, grounded, de-stressed, energized, effortless breathing
Disgust	Nausea, repulsion, distaste, discomfort, intolerance, offensiveness, loathing, contamination, revulsion, disdain, abhorrence, contempt, aversion	Vomiting, gag reflex, sweating, coldness, goosebumps, loss of appetite, grimacing, watery eyes, holding breath, sensitivity to sensory input, recoiling

- What emotions come up on repeat?

- When checking out your emotional response to a situation, ask yourself, 'Do my emotions line up with this situation? How would I intellectually *expect* someone to respond emotionally to this? Does that ring true for me too? If not, why not? Is something getting in the way of my authentic emotional expression?'

Perhaps complete your own table of emotions and sensations as detailed above, so you can get to know your own emotional language and how it's expressed through the body. Consider the journal prompts above and really get to know yourself on this emotional level to set your healing in motion. Whilst we'll all respond differently to situations, if we have developed a maladaptive emotional response based on experiences from the past and it's impacting us in a negative way, then we need an awareness of this so that we can understand and learn a more beneficial way of being.

It's also helpful to link this emotional awareness with the specific events you wish to work on from the past, and perhaps connect this with your memory of the event. Decipher whether this is generating a lower frequency energy that could be detrimentally impacting your life; for example, you could say, 'When I think back to the day my girlfriend hit me, I notice I feel shame, embarrassment, helplessness and anger. I feel this in my body as muscle tension in my hands, a clenched jaw and a fast heartbeat.' Gather together a number of the incidents you'd like to clear, noticing how much is unresolved, and gain an awareness of what you're carrying energetically too.

Remember your physical illnesses and problems have an underlying emotional aspect. In the previous chapter we listened to the voice of the body as it expressed itself through pain. Now ask yourself, 'What emotions are connected to this physical problem or life issue? How does it make me feel now? How do I emotionally relate to having this illness or to experiencing this difficulty in my life?' What was happening in my life when this physical problem appeared? How does this relate to how I was feeling then? If that illness, body part or situation was a feeling, what would it be?

By exploring the emotional elements intertwined with challenges at the physical level, you can gain a deeper understanding of their interplay and potentially uncover valuable insights about these difficulties and your underlying core need. This can be helpful when addressing, processing and releasing them.

We'll come to this soon, but first it might be handy to know a couple of techniques that can help direct you to those roots.

Applied Kinesiology

Applied Kinesiology (AK), also referred to as muscle testing, is a holistic practice used by some healthcare providers to assess the body's overall health, diagnose medical conditions and suggest appropriate treatments. The theory behind AK is that muscles are linked to other parts of the body through a network of neurological pathways, and that muscle weakness when testing may indicate an underlying imbalance or dysfunction within the body. This imbalance may be related to factors such as physical or emotional stress, nutrient deficiencies, allergies, toxins or other issues that disrupt the body's natural balance.

The mechanism by which a muscle goes weak during AK testing isn't fully understood and is a subject of debate among practitioners and researchers. Some theories suggest that it may relate to changes in the muscle's electrical activity, the nervous system's response to stress, a disruption to the body's energy flow, or a phenomenon known as 'neurological inhibition', where the brain temporarily reduces the strength of certain muscles following conflicting signals from different parts of the body. The theory is that AK testing can reveal these neurological inhibitions and thus identify underlying imbalances or dysfunctions.

Whilst there is a lot of anecdotal evidence in support of this approach, research studies haven't consistently demonstrated the effectiveness or scientific validity of AK, so it's important to approach it with a critical mindset. That said, it *is* recognized by the Complementary and National Healthcare Council (CNHC) and thousands of practitioners use it effectively on a daily basis, so this is why I offer to you an awareness of it here, so you can experiment for yourself.

This technique usually has another person doing the testing for you, so it can be a little challenging when using it by yourself; however, your confidence and accuracy will improve with practice. The main priority is to nurture a neutral state of mind with unbiased intent when doing it. Your thinking mind will pop in and try to predict or influence the outcome if you're not in the correct headspace, so please do be mindful of that. A little meditation beforehand can help you to overcome this, as can approaching it from a place where you're not invested in the outcome. Imagine you're working with a stranger.

I'm introducing this approach *only* as a way of helping you to connect with your *inner*-tuition and what you need to heal. By focusing on specific life events from your journal, potentially blocked emotions, harmful beliefs, etc., you can establish what the body needs to clear in order to come back to balance. Presenting these scenarios as questions and using muscle testing alongside them will help you to find the emotional energy from these unprocessed experiences that is still stuck. Once you have identified it, you can go on to clear and process it using Emotional Freedom Technique (EFT) (*page 187*).

Applied Kinesiology

Preparation

▲ **Neutrality**: Release any attachment to a particular outcome.

▲ **Clarity**: Be clear about what you're testing. Know what a strong/weak response indicates.

▲ **Centred**: Connect with the present moment and with the body via a few deep breaths.

▲ **Cleanse energy**: We all pick up energetic debris as we go through our daily lives, much like our houses pick up dust. So, first do a body scan (*page 44*) and release any tension in the body. Bring in a ball of white light above your head and imagine the energy showering down on you, just as if you were in a physical shower. Send out the intention that any energy that's not your own will be washed away, and see the 'shower' doing just that. Allow any energetic debris you've collected to simply swirl away down an imaginary plughole.

▲ **Recall energy**: In the same way that you pick up energy from other people and places, you may leave bits of your own energy behind, so send out the intention to call back any of your own energy that's been misplaced. Feel it returning to you, allowing you to feel whole.

Now we may begin.

There are a number of ways you can use muscle testing, most often related to pushing down your outstretched arm or pulling apart interlocking fingers. Here I will show you the standing test. It should be the easiest to follow, as it uses the whole body. What works well for one person can be less effective for another, though, so if this doesn't resonate with you, do check out other versions online.

The Standing Test

From the discoveries made by Dr Candace Pert, we now know that our nervous system responds to our thoughts and emotions, influencing our body's movements through its connection to the brain. Our unconscious mind, which operates independently of logic and reasoning, has a natural inclination towards what it perceives as positive or truthful, and a tendency to reject what it deems negative or untrue. This technique is based on this premise, so when you ask questions whilst standing in a relaxed position, the body will involuntarily sway forwards or backwards, indicating agreement or disagreement with your statements. Words are effectively just energy, so the body acts as a pendulum, showing whether it resonates with your words or not.

Directions:

1. Set your intention to access your body as an instrument for communication. Stand up straight with your feet shoulder-width apart, ensuring both feet point directly forwards. Bend your knees slightly, so they're not locked and place your hands down at your sides. Imagine roots going from your feet down into the ground.

2. Close your eyes (if it's safe to do so), drop your awareness into the body and take a few deep breaths.

3. Now you're ready to test for accuracy to ensure this bodily response reflects a true representation of what is asked. Say out loud: 'Show me a "yes"...' and wait. You should notice the body involuntarily leans slightly forwards in response, showing you that it resonates with what you're saying.

4. Next, try the same with: 'Show me a "no"...' This time the body should involuntarily lean slightly backwards, showing you it rejects or is repelled by what you're saying.

5. You're now ready to gain deeper insight into your life by exploring what needs to be cleared from your past, by asking questions relevant to what you have learnt as you have worked your way through this book.

As well as identifying emotional blocks, this process can be applied to test for blockages in the mind. You can ask about anything you feel needs to be healed, such as:

- Blockages from childhood, ancestral trauma, trauma in the womb, difficulties from past or parallel lives

- Beliefs, thought patterns and past programming that could be holding you back

- Established conflicts to healing, or secondary gains of remaining where you are and resisting change

- Blocks to realizing your aspirations and fulfilling your purpose

You might experience some personal variations to the standard forwards or backwards responses – you may lean from left to right, or sway diagonally for example. What's important to know is what response is consistently communicating accurate answers to you. If you're getting opposite responses, however, with backwards for 'yes', it's most likely because your energy isn't balanced enough, so it might be beneficial to do some grounding exercises as given in the previous chapter. Other conditions that can interfere include dehydration, fatigue, hunger and blood sugar imbalance. Otherwise the interference probably centres around doubt, either about yourself or about the muscle testing itself. In this instance, you may need to work on this before continuing. You could release any blocks around this with EFT, which we will come to in a moment.

Pendulum Dowsing

An alternative to using the body to identify areas to work on is using a pendulum to connect with and receive answers from your *inner*-tuition. The movement of the pendulum serves as a tangible way to receive guidance from within.

You may or may not be familiar with this tool, but a pendulum can be any weighted object that hangs freely from a cord or chain. I personally tend to use crystal pendulums, as due to their molecular structure they form a unique energetic bond, amplifying intention and enhancing the resonance and clarity of communication from a higher Self that so often goes unheard. A crystal isn't some inert piece of rock worn by gullible hippies; each type has distinct energetic properties and vibrations that can impact the energy field around them. Quartz, for example, is often used in modern technology. It's found in computer chips, smartphones, even the Hale Telescope, but what's interesting to note is you've probably been wearing one for much of your life. Have a look at your watch. Chances are, it's the electrical energy from a quartz crystal that's keeping its time – perhaps crystals aren't so woo-woo after all!

There are many crystal pendulums to choose from, each with its own energetic frequency and qualities, so you could perhaps choose one that corresponds with your intention, or one that relates to your ailment or particular situation, or even with the level of the Self you're working with (*see below*).

Level of Self	Suggested Crystals
Body	Jasper, clear quartz, bloodstone, golden healer
Emotions	Malachite, citrine, lepidolite, carnelian
Mind	Obsidian, fluorite, smoky quartz, tiger's eye
Intuition	Moonstone, labradorite, amethyst, lapis lazuli
Relationship Self/Other	Green aventurine, rose quartz, rhodonite, sodalite

You could also just simply choose whichever one you feel drawn to – even a simple clear quartz would be a perfect all-rounder for this work.

Using a pendulum to gain answers about what you need to release from the body, emotions, mind, energetic field and relationships is probably seen to be a little far-fetched, especially as many people incorrectly believe a pendulum is just a tool used to speak with the dead. I personally prefer to use this technique over kinesiology and find it a wonderful tool for gaining insight and clarity. We will be using it to access our inner guidance here so we can find those answers we may struggle to access at a conscious level.

Setting the intention is the first step towards achieving any goal, and the same goes for using a pendulum. If you're looking to connect with the energy of your deceased loved ones, then yes, you can use this to communicate with them. Similarly, if you're seeking guidance from spirit guides, angels or other elemental beings, you can use this as a means of connecting with them also. However, in this particular instance, your intention is to focus on connecting with your higher Self to gain valuable insight into what needs healing from the past and what direction to take in the future. You may programme different intentions for different crystals or pendulums.

Using a Pendulum

Once you've chosen your pendulum, it's important to cleanse and programme it before dowsing.

Cleansing

To cleanse it, try:

▲ moon bathing, sun bathing (if safe for that crystal)

▲ running water (not for crystals ending in 'ite', as they may become toxic, dissolve or break apart)

- ▲ smudging

- ▲ Reiki

- ▲ sound vibration

- ▲ a saltwater bath

Programming

Directions:

1. Hold the crystal between your cupped hands and direct your awareness to it, focusing on the connection between your energy and your pendulum.

2. Clear your mind and take a few deep breaths.

3. Set your intention for using the pendulum as clearly as possible.

4. Hold the crystal up to your third eye chakra (located between your eyebrows) and visualize your intention or desired outcome entering the crystal. You may also choose to speak your intention out loud into the crystal.

Dowsing

Directions:

1. Sit in a comfortable position holding your pendulum out in front of you. The chain should hang down over the top of the forefinger on your dominant hand, with your thumb securing it in place. Keep your elbow close to the body to help with stability.

2. Bring the pendulum to a place of stillness, above the palm of your other open hand, and relax!

3. Start by finding how the pendulum will respond by saying, 'Show me your... "yes"/"no"/"maybe"/"I don't know."' Wait for the pendulum to start moving with each instruction; it might move from side to side, forwards to backwards, clockwise to anti-clockwise. Make note of the direction it moves in for all the responses.

You must follow all the steps above whenever you work with a new crystal, as they all respond differently. A 'no' with one pendulum might actually be a 'yes' on another, and vice versa.

Now you know what each answer looks like, take some time to ask questions you already know the answer to, so you can start building up trust.

It can take time to understand how your individual pendulum communicates, so be patient. The more time you devote to this practice, the better you'll get!

Once confident, you can start asking questions to direct your healing, to clarify what's negatively impacting you and to ask for life guidance.

//

When using the pendulum or muscle testing, keep your questions in a yes/no format, and make them simple and specific, so you can get a clear answer. In particular, it might be helpful to find what's blocking you from finding the fulfilling future you desire. Really get to the root of what you specifically need to release; for example, 'Is my lethargy and depressed mood caused by unprocessed emotions from my miscarriage?' or 'Do I have anger I need to release before I will get pregnant again?' or 'Do I need to work on an energetic connection to call in a baby?' Questions like these really help to give a specific answer to what needs healing and on what level – physically, emotionally, mentally, spiritually, relationally. Then you can just keep asking questions until you have more of an insight into the difficulties you're carrying so you can process them and clear any blocks using techniques that work with releasing this emotional energy.

Emotional Freedom Technique

Emotional Freedom Technique (EFT), also referred to as tapping therapy or a psychological form of acupuncture, is a powerful yet simple therapeutic tool that stimulates a series of acupressure points through tapping whilst simultaneously focusing on issues that need to be healed or cleared. This technique works by rebalancing the meridians, the network of energy pathways, and enables us to release and transform uncomfortable emotions, thinking patterns and beliefs that may be negatively impacting our health and wellbeing. It's not necessarily the memory or trauma itself, but what happens to the energy system in relation to that trauma that causes the emotions that can end up stuck.

I first trained in this technique in my early twenties; however, I never used it with my clients because it seemed so bizarre and, quite frankly, unprofessional. There was no way I was going to advocate tapping set points along some 'imaginary' energy system. My dismissal of this approach meant it was years before I read the vast amount of research that showed its benefits.

It was actually witnessing the transformative impact it had on my daughter Lyla that led me to re-evaluate this tool. She was about seven years old at the time and deeply unhappy at school, crying every morning and night, anxious about going in. She was somehow unable to access the language to verbalize why she was struggling so much, and I was at a loss as to how to help – that was, until as a last resort we did a round of EFT. Within a matter of minutes, there was a tsunami of words and emotions – it was as if the tapping had suddenly opened the floodgates – and all the difficult scenarios Lyla was facing were expressed in an instant. It was nothing short of miraculous and pretty amazing to see.

It's intriguing that despite its pseudoscientific appearance, there's actually quite a substantial body of evidence that demonstrates the effectiveness of EFT for a variety of psychological and physiological conditions. In a 2022 systematic review of 56 randomized controlled trials and eight meta-analyses, EFT was found to be an effective treatment for psychological conditions such as anxiety, depression, phobias and post-traumatic stress disorder (PTSD); physiological issues such as pain, insomnia and autoimmune conditions; professional and sports performance enhancement; and reducing the biological markers of stress, such as cortisol.[8]

Randomized controlled trials (RCTs) assessing the effectiveness of EFT for many conditions haven't only shown encouraging outcomes, they have also indicated that few treatment sessions are required, that treatment is effective whether delivered in person or virtually, and that symptom improvements persist over time. It's also reported that there are no adverse effects from using EFT and it can be used both on a self-help basis and as a primary evidence-based treatment.[9] Not bad going for a bit of tapping! It's not surprising that its use in primary care settings as a reliable and effective treatment continues to grow, so much so that it's even recommended in the guidelines from the National Institute for Health and Care Excellence (NICE) for further research as a treatment for PTSD.[10]

So, you now have the language and awareness to connect with and express your emotions, but how do you decide what stuck feelings or events need to be released? You may be thinking that it'll take forever to clear and heal all the things that have come up for you, but in reality there is usually a core memory at the root, which if processed and cleared, helps to release the other memory layers connected via that vibrational frequency. For example, my client 'Dan'* felt his inability to commit to his current partner was due to his previous partners having left him; however, his fear of commitment actually linked back to his father having been the sole survivor of a car crash where he lost both his parents and a sibling. Instead of working through each relationship abandonment one by one, we worked to heal and clear the meaning and emotional charge of the root experience, which then released the rest and enabled him to commit more deeply and break the cycle of disconnect.

---

*   Names have been changed to maintain confidentiality.

Emotional Freedom Technique

By exploring your emotions and utilizing techniques such as muscle testing and pendulum dowsing, you may have gained some valuable insight into what past emotions might be impacting your present and your future. Now, let's look at releasing them, using EFT.

Step 1: Identifying the Issue

1. **Labelling**: First start with an unprocessed experience or illness you have chosen to work with and give it a 'title', for example, 'The day my dad left home.' If you have chosen something from before your birth, whether generational trauma or something from a past life, treat it in the same way.

2. **Identifying the emotions**: Bring to mind the experience you're processing and identify which emotions are present – you'll be focusing on these during the procedure.

3. **Rating the intensity**: On a scale of 0-10, rate how intense the emotional charge feels for you (10 being the strongest). If you can locate where you 'feel' it in the body, also take note of that. It's good practice to have an idea of your starting point so you can gauge your progress. If you don't feel an emotional charge right now, that's fine too.

4. **Acknowledging the event**: Allow yourself to remember the experience or situation briefly. Write down the thoughts, memories and beliefs that resonate with this situation so we can then work to restructure them in the next chapter on the mental level of Self, but also so you can add them to the processing here.

The mind usually searches to make meaning before it can let go of something, but that's not a necessary component of this technique. Remember all the levels are connected with one another energetically, and it's the energy we're working with, hence why this approach will work with past lives and inherited ancestral patterns, and why it worked with

Lyla, even though I had no idea what was bothering her. We're effectively releasing the glue that binds it all together, so just work with what you do know, and with a positive intent, and know that this change is coming.

Step 2: The Tapping Sequence

The first thing you need to know is where the points are. See the diagram below.

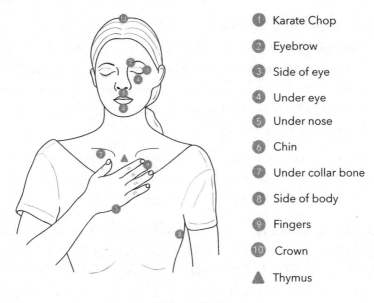

1. Karate Chop
2. Eyebrow
3. Side of eye
4. Under eye
5. Under nose
6. Chin
7. Under collar bone
8. Side of body
9. Fingers
10. Crown
▲ Thymus

Tapping Points

The karate chop (KC) point is located at the centre of the fleshy part of the outside of your non-dominant hand – where you would deliver a karate chop. This is where we begin the sequence with a 'set-up' statement.

The set-up is a process used to start each round of tapping. Whilst *continuously* tapping the KC point, you let your system know what you're trying to address.

To do this, you state the 'title' of problem, alongside a phrase that brings about a sense of accepting yourself despite it. It usually goes something like, 'Even though [insert title of problem], I deeply and completely love and accept myself.' Now, the second part of that statement can be a bit much for some, so I will often ask people to focus on something they know to be true about themselves that they value, or even simply stating that they're okay anyway.

Some alternative set-up statements could be:

▲ 'Even though my father abandoned me, I'm a deeply loyal person.'

▲ 'Even though my body is failing me and I'm in tremendous pain, I'm okay.'

▲ 'Even though I'm frightened to leave the house, I love and accept myself.'

You have a little flexibility when designing your set-up phrase, but be sure to include both parts.

State this three times whilst tapping the KC point and focusing on the issue.

Then, with a fairly firm pressure, we move on to tap the acupressure points with our fingertips, around 7–10 times (no need to count), in the following sequence:

1. At the beginning of the eyebrow, just above and to one side of the nose.

2. On the eye socket bone at the outside corner of the eye.

3. Along the bottom of the eye socket bone in line with your pupil.

4. Between the bottom of your nose and the top of your upper lip.

5. Midway between the point of your chin and the bottom of your lower lip.

6. Just under the collar bone, approximately one inch down and two inches left/right of the top of the breastbone (where you would knot a tie). There is often a tender indentation there.

7. Under the arm on the side of the body, about four inches below the armpit.

8. Fingers of non-dominant hand – edge of nail bed on thumb, first finger, then middle finger – all on the side closest to the body. The point on the ring finger is the opposite side, but again you're tapping on the finger at the edge of the nail. The little finger is back to the side closest to the body.

9. Back to karate chop point.

10. Crown of the head; this is the intersecting point if you were to draw a line from one ear to the other, and another line from your nose to the back of your neck. There are lots of nerve endings here, so use all your fingertips.

It doesn't matter which side of the body you use – you can even use both at the same time if you like.

As you tap on each point, say a couple of words that relate to what you need to clear. Try using a mix of thoughts, emotions and physical sensations in your descriptions, along with more specific details of the event, such as the environment, something negative that was said, a smell that triggers you, etc. For example, you might tap on one point and say, 'My fear of failure,' the next, 'The panic rising from my stomach,' the next, 'Mum said I was a loser,' and the next, 'The humiliation.' Dig deep – it's important you focus on the worst elements of the situation. You're bringing it all out into the open so you can process and release it. I know it seems counter-intuitive, or perhaps even a little scary or painful, to focus on the negative, but make sure you stay with the tapping, and the emotional charge will reduce.

If you don't know or remember the details of the event, or if it's a past-life or generational experience, you can use a set-up like 'Even though something happened when I was a child and I don't remember the details, I deeply love and accept myself,' or 'Even though my anger comes from generations past, I'm okay anyway.' Remember the muscle testing or pendulum would have helped you to ascertain this anger as being related to events before your birth.

The tapping-point phrases for these unknown situations could remain generic, along the lines of 'The details from that experience' or 'The harm that was caused.'

You can even take the metaphorical insight given by the body and work with that. You might not know exactly what it's connected to, but it will still clear the energy. For example, I know why my legs would collapse as I walked, but if I hadn't made the connection with all the trauma I was carrying, I could still tap on 'My legs giving way' or 'I can't carry any more' or 'The pain trapped inside' and this would help with clearing what was behind it anyway.

It can even help to imagine the difficulty you're working on as a movie, using the set-up phrase as the film title and the tapping points as the individual scenes. This approach can be particularly helpful with overwhelming events you may feel you still need some distance from, such as trauma.

Step 3: The Check-in

Now you've completed one round of EFT, take a deep breath, close your eyes and check in with yourself.

Tune back into the energy of the experience you were working with and rate the intensity of emotional charge again on a scale of 0–10.

Notice what's changed and whether the physical sensation or the emotional rating has gone down at all. Some people notice an immediate shift with just one round, whilst others will need many, but there need be no judgement.

Just take a moment to check your original set-up and amend as necessary, so you can begin a new round.

It can be a bit like peeling an onion – once you get to the end of a tapping round, a new focus can be revealed. Remember, different situations can be connected energetically, so don't be surprised if other scenarios come through for healing. You might have started the process believing you were working on your heartbreak at having separated from your wife and end up working on that time you saw your dog get run over when you were four years old. Just trust in the process and repeat the rounds until you feel some relief.

Note also that it's not unheard-of for the intensity of the emotion to increase; this is actually a good sign, as the imbalanced energy is mobilizing and coming to the surface to be healed. Make sure you continue tapping through any surge in symptoms as you need to get through to the other side. Only stop when the intensity has reduced.

You'll know instinctively when you've cleared your situation, as your emotional charge will have reduced right down. For those of you who are still a little disconnected or uncertain, you can use the pendulum dowsing or muscle testing to check – literally asking if you have cleared the emotion or if the experience is still influencing you in a negative way.

There really is no need to rush this, and you may require a little time for the processing to be completed, so a tapping break might be essential before you start seeing results. Remember, healing needs time – you can't just expect a few minutes of tapping will clear things straight away. Patience and persistence are key.

Step 4: The Closing Round

If you've processed your experience fully, or you've decided to take a tapping break, it can be helpful to close with a positive round by giving the body positive emotions and affirmations to put in the place of what you've released.

Here you just simply install some positive or peaceful phrases in exactly the same sequence as before, remembering to focus on the feeling of these suggestions as you do so.

You can also reflect on where you feel you're at now the event has been processed and install what that now means about you, how you now feel, what you would rather identify as, etc... Install that!

Thymus Tapping

Another way to install this is by tapping on your thymus gland to send the positive vibration through your whole system. This can be found in the centre of the chest (*as detailed on page 188*). Remember to breathe deeply as you do so, and set the intention that you're sending the vibration of [*insert positive emotion*] through all the levels of the Self.

//

You can make peace with your past by systematically working through the origins of those pre-programmed behaviours, difficult memories, addictions, painful relationships, traumas and physical and mental illnesses plaguing the present, by using EFT to permanently remove the emotional charge.

Remember, you don't need to complete this work alone. Healing can be really profound when done through a therapeutic relationship, so do invest in professional support if you feel you might benefit from it. The premise of this book is that armed with the right tools and awareness you can be your own best healer, but there are many situations where healing through the relationship with another person, therapeutic or not, is a fundamental part of the process.

However you choose to move forwards, you now need to address the impact of what you carry at the mental level of the Self.

CHAPTER 12
THE MIND MATTERS

Do you ever wonder what goes on inside the minds of other people? I know I do – that's one of the reasons I became a psychologist, I suppose. But how about your own mind? How often do you pay attention to that? To that constant stream of thoughts your mind generates? According to a 2020 study using fMRI brain scanning to observe the transition from one thought to another, the average human may have around 6,200 thoughts per day, the contents of which may be much more important than you might realize.[1]

In his book *The Biology of Belief*, Dr Bruce Lipton presents scientific discoveries relating to the biochemical effects of the brain's functioning and demonstrates how *all* the cells of our body are affected by our thoughts.[2] He suggests that switching to a more constructive outlook could positively impact our emotions, our health and our life. Dr Candace Pert talks of this also, and explains how the complex interconnections between our physical, emotional and mental states can be attributed to the neuropeptides produced by nerve cells in the brain.[3] These neuropeptides create a sophisticated information network that communicates with receptors throughout the body.

This interplay between our thoughts and body was also demonstrated by Masaru Emoto, a Japanese researcher and author who claimed that his experiments showed that positive and negative words, thoughts and emotions changed the molecular structure of water.[4] When water was exposed to positive thoughts and words, it formed beautiful, intricate crystals, while when it was exposed to negative stimuli, it formed distorted, chaotic structures.

Emoto went on to propose that as the human body has a high percentage of water, such a structural shift could positively or negatively influence human cells and tissues. If you look at these images, it'll make you think twice before saying how much you 'hate your body' or repeatedly telling yourself how 'ill' or 'stupid' you are.

There is some controversy surrounding these research findings, but one thing's for sure: If you're in an unfavourable environment, either externally (people around you) or internally (self-talk), where you're constantly exposed to negative, judgemental or unkind words, you're likely to be detrimentally impacted. So, why wouldn't that affect you at every level of the Self and in every cell of the body – it's all connected after all?

In addition to the health conditions associated with stress and trauma, research has also shown negative self-talk to be associated with a relapse of anxiety and depression.[5] The cynicism and hostility that are likely to unfold under such conditions have also been linked to a greater risk of dementia,[6] heart disease and stroke,[7] diabetes,[8] heart attacks[9] and inflammatory conditions relating to stress.[10] This is also true in reverse, of course, with research showing that positive cognitions generate beneficial psychological states,[11] enhance emotional regulation,[12] increase sports and academic performance,[13] and improve depression,[14] anxiety and stress.[15]

If we adhere to the premise that we're a unified energetic system of consciousness with interconnected thoughts, feelings, emotions, behaviours, actions and interactions, it does make sense that the thoughts we generate have a significant impact on the course of our life, our health, our relationships and our wellbeing. It has even been suggested that our

DNA can be affected both by negative and positive thoughts, beliefs and emotions,[16] as although epigenetics has revealed that the environment controls the expression of these genes, it's more specifically our *perception* of this environment. Remember, what impacts one level of the Self impacts them all, so it's essential to be mindful of the thoughts we generate and ensure they line up with the outcomes we want to create.

REFRAMING THINKING PATTERNS

Are *you* actively aware of the outcomes you wish to create in your life, and are your thoughts in alignment with this? Or are you passively allowing your subconscious programming to do the work for you?

The Subconscious Mind

Unlike the conscious mind, which involves the thoughts we're aware of at any given moment, the subconscious mind operates *below* the surface of our awareness and is responsible for making decisions and performing tasks without any conscious thought. Driving a car is often given as a great example of this, where steps like changing gear, checking mirrors and stopping in an emergency have become subconscious and run on autopilot. In the same way, it's your subconscious mind that's responsible for getting you to a familiar destination when you 'suddenly' find you've arrived with no recall of the journey. Well, that's a pretty good analogy for how many of us live our lives. If we're not fully present, perhaps stressing about the future or replaying the past, then we're not in the driving seat of our life or conscious of many of the choices, thoughts and actions we are taking – we've defaulted to a pre-programmed subconscious and so have little say in where we end up!

Our subconscious mind does have a positive function – it takes over routine tasks and automates processes in the name of efficiency, thus freeing up headspace for the conscious mind – but in addition to being the source of our automatic behaviours and habits, it is also believed to store our deeper beliefs and values, which can be difficult to access or change without conscious intervention, or the use of tools such as meditation, hypnotherapy, creative visualization and EFT. These beliefs and values form a part of our reality, impacting our decisions and behaviours without our knowledge. For example, if you were raised with the belief that money was hard to come by, you may find it challenging to manifest financial abundance in your life, even if you consciously desire and value wealth.

Here are some common examples of how the subconscious mind can show up and influence your life:

- **Emotions**: The subconscious mind stores emotional memories that can be activated by certain stimuli unconsciously, triggering sudden mood swings or overwhelm.

- **Phobias**: Often triggered by specific objects or situations that are rooted in subconscious programming, such as a traumatic experience from childhood or conditioning from having observed others.

- **Relationship patterns**: If your parents had a dysfunctional relationship, that imprint remains in the subconscious and you may unknowingly seek out a partner who exhibits similar patterns of behaviour.

- **Self-talk**: Negative internal dialogue, such as 'I'm not good enough' or 'I'll never succeed', can be a result of subconscious programming from past events and can limit your potential.

- **Habits**: Repeated exposure to a particular stimulus leads to conditioning – an automatic learned response is created to make it easier/more efficient for us to perform in the future.

Do you ever notice how often your subconscious mind is taking the driving seat in your life, and are you even aware of the negative impact it could be having? What if you were to shift to a more conscious approach and deliberately start to shape your own future? If you're reading this book, it's likely you're looking to make some positive changes in your life, and that's exactly what we're here to do. So, let's dive into some practical strategies to help you purge the past from this subconscious programming and start consciously calling in your desired future.

Neuroplasticity

The brain is in a constant state of change – it's either busy creating new pathways or it's strengthening those that already exist. Brain plasticity, also known as neuroplasticity, is a term that refers to the brain's capacity to change and adapt as a result of experience. Early researchers believed that neurogenesis, the creation of new neurons, stopped shortly after birth. They assumed the brain was a 'non-renewable organ' with a finite number of cells that slowly died as we aged. We now understand, however, that the brain possesses the remarkable ability to create new connections, reorganize pathways and even grow new neurons.

Unlike computers, which are built as fixed hardware structures and receive periodic software upgrades, our brains, in addition to receiving software updates (as a result of our experiences, adapted belief systems and exposure to new frequencies of energetic input), also receive hardware updates. When we learn something new, the brain itself changes, rewiring neuronal connections to adapt to these new circumstances. This happens automatically on a daily basis but can also be consciously encouraged in a way that can help us to construct a new life that can remain, because what fires together, wires together!

So if you're repeatedly doing, thinking, feeling and believing the same things each and every day, then they're going to get recorded in the subconscious mind. Whether for your benefit or not, those neural pathways simply become stronger and stronger, reaffirming the life that already exists – the one that was generated in the past! So, if you're wanting to learn, be or do something new, then you need to switch from the autopilot and challenge your brain to make some new connections. The conscious repetition of new desired beliefs, emotions, habits and actions etches out and deepens new pathways, until they become stronger than the old ones. Like a redirected river, these new connections will flow easily and effortlessly, whilst the old flow will dry up!

Subconscious re-programming starts with deciding what you want, something we will focus on in the final chapter of this book. Right now, we're going to bring into your conscious awareness the programming you need to release.

If the Self-connection quiz revealed that your thinking mind is an area in need of your attention, whether you're preoccupied by your thoughts or detached from them, the key to finding balance is *presence*. If you've been consistently following a daily practice that involves the tools to promote a peaceful present, then I'm sure you'll have found some balance within the thinking mind already. The three-minute breathing space in particular will bring to your conscious attention the kind of thoughts you're having, and based on everything you've learnt up to this point, you're more likely to be aware now of how such thoughts could be detrimentally impacting your life.

REWRITING THE SCRIPT

Thoughts aren't facts, yet we live our lives as if they were. They're subjective mental processes that are shaped by our beliefs, emotions and past experiences, and involve our individual interpretation, evaluation and perception of information. Here are some of the common distorted thought patterns we often mindlessly swallow as the 'truth'. Take a look, I'm sure you'll recognize some of them:

- **Catastrophizing**: Anticipating the worst possible outcome of a situation and blowing it out of proportion. This type of thinking can lead to excessive worry and anxiety.

- **Overgeneralization:** Drawing broad conclusions based on a single incident or piece of evidence. This type of thinking can lead to negative and unrealistic beliefs about oneself or others.

- **Personalization:** Assuming negative events or situations reflect your personal shortcomings or faults, even with no supporting evidence. This thinking can lead to low self-esteem, shame and self-doubt.

- **Mind-reading:** Assuming you know what others are thinking or feeling, without any evidence to support it. This type of thinking can lead to misunderstandings and conflicts in relationships.

- **All-or-nothing thinking:** Seeing situations as black and white, with no shades of grey in between. This type of thinking can lead to a narrow and inflexible view of the world.

- **Emotional reasoning:** Believing your emotions accurately reflect reality and allowing them to guide your thoughts and behaviour. This type of thinking can lead to impulsive decisions and irrational behaviour.

- **Mental filtering:** Ignoring information we don't expect to see or believe to be true. And seeking only evidence that confirms our beliefs, whilst filtering out anything to the contrary. This can lead to feelings of depression, anxiety and low self-esteem as negative experiences or failures are magnified.

- **Discounting the positive:** Focusing only on negative aspects of a situation or experience and discounting or ignoring positive aspects. This type of thinking can lead to feelings of hopelessness and despair.

We need to catch thought distortions such as these, as they can actually contribute to various mental health conditions. They will show up in our everyday life, so it's important we're able to identify and challenge them. Keep them in mind as you work through the exercises in this chapter and notice where they're making an appearance. Before you get to challenge them, we first need to unblock any more general beliefs you may be carrying that have the potential to get in the way of your healing.

Blocks to Healing

If you believe you can or if
you believe you can't... you're right.

HENRY FORD

When someone believes something they do or take will improve their health, an improvement is often seen. This is a well-documented healing phenomenon called the placebo effect.[17] The same is true of the nocebo effect, which is when negative beliefs and expectations about a treatment or condition can worsen symptoms and health outcomes.[18,19] So if you hold beliefs that could hinder your healing, such as believing you can't release difficulties and heal from your past, or you can't generate a new future for yourself, then chances are, you'll be correct.

Psychological factors such as this can have a massive influence on your life in general, as well as play a crucial role in your healing. Take the case of Sam Londe in 1974[20]: diagnosed with oesophageal cancer, he died a few weeks later. This wasn't deemed unusual back then, but his autopsy revealed there was actually no cancer in his oesophagus, just a few spots on his liver and one on his lung. None were enough to kill him. It's believed that his fear and belief he had fatal cancer triggered the nocebo effect and may have actually contributed to his decline in health and eventual death.

I believe a big part of the reason I've been able to heal myself from such a significant number of serious health conditions relates to this, as I've never fully identified as an unwell person – my beliefs have helped me to heal. By not fully embracing the persona of someone with these illnesses, I was never fully aligned with keeping them. Now let me be clear, I'm not talking about denial here, which in and of itself can start the cycle of disconnection that brings about an issue or illness. I was very conscious of the illnesses, but I viewed them as visitors and chose to remind myself that they weren't permitted to stay.

Consider the people who win millions in the lottery and then find themselves destitute a year later. They were never fully in alignment with the identity of a multi-millionaire across all the levels of the Self.

I always knew I didn't need to keep the illnesses; I just needed to take the lessons and could then choose to heal, part of which was knowing, believing and identifying as someone whole and healed. I'm here to show you how to do that too. Whether it's poor health, limited wealth or a rocky relationship, the process is always the same – we release the old behaviours, the old feelings, thoughts and energy of what we want to release and bring in the elements that relate to what we want to call in. This is the main philosophy behind my release and re-programming method.

So let's come back and check those beliefs lurking in your mind that might well be blocking you from healing the past, generating change and enjoying that favourable future. I have indicated six main categories in the table opposite that will be likely to relate to some of your blocks:

Blocks	Beliefs preventing healing/change
Desire *'I don't want to recover/ change/heal.'*	At a subconscious level, you may not wish to recover/ change/heal due to the positive aspects of your situation (secondary gains). *e.g. 'I feel more loved when I'm ill, people notice me more.'*
Fear *'Change is unsafe.'*	Resisting change and the vulnerability required to heal or recover can get in the way if you can't step out of your comfort zone. *e.g. 'I must stick with what I know or my life might get worse.'*
Trust *'It's impossible for me to heal.'*	You're sceptical about the possibility that healing or change can occur or, more specifically, whether it's possible for you! *e.g. 'I've been stuck like this for years, nothing and no one can help me.'*
Readiness *'I'm not ready to recover/ change/heal.'*	Your problem is so deeply ingrained in your sense of Self that you're not ready to let it go – it's a part of who you are; it's your identity. *e.g. 'I'm a loser in love – always have been, always will be.'*
Worthiness *'I'm unworthy of healing/ recovery.'*	You've had multiple failures/setbacks when attempting to heal/change so feel powerless or unworthy of progress. *e.g. 'Positive things never happen for someone like me.'*
Ability *'I don't know how to recover/change/ heal.'*	You don't feel you have the ability or the 'know-how' to be able to heal or change – you're just not capable of recovery. *e.g. 'I'm not able to heal or change my life – I'm stuck!'*

Releasing the Blocks to Healing

Identifying Negative Thoughts

Take a moment to connect with any limiting beliefs you have about your ability to heal or to facilitate change in your life and, using the table and categories on the previous page as a guide, write in your journal what core beliefs, and perhaps even sub-beliefs, could be blocking your way. Remember to look out for any cognitive distortions!

Reviewing Readiness

Establish whether you're ready to let these blocks go. You can do this using your *inner*-tuition:

▲ **Sitting in the power**: Asking your higher Self, guides, ancestors, the Universe, whatever you relate to: 'Am I ready to let go of [*insert the block you're checking here*]?' and wait for a response – it will be spoken in your mind, seen as an image or movie, felt as a sensation in the body, or you'll 'just kind of know'.

▲ **Checking in with your heart intelligence**: Put your hands on your heart, connect with the energy in the heart chakra, and say, 'My heart, am I ready to let go of [*insert the block you're checking here*]?' You'll get a very clear 'yes' or 'no'.

▲ **Using kinesiology or a pendulum**: If you're still strengthening your *inner*-tuition, then you can use kinesiology as detailed previously (*page 178*) or ask your questions via the pendulum (*page 182*). Just do what works best for you.

If the response shows you're not yet ready to release these blocks, then in the same way ask if there is more to learn from this belief before you can let it go. If 'no', then you're ready to continue to the next step, and if 'yes', ask if there is an unprocessed experience that created this belief that needs releasing first. If that's the case, then use EFT (*page 187*) to process this experience.

Challenging Negative Thoughts

Question the validity of these beliefs and look for concrete evidence or a factual basis for them. Are they based on past experiences, societal conditioning or assumptions? Are they cognitive distortions? Challenge the assumptions and biases that could underpin them.

Seeking Alternative Perspectives

What else could be going on here? What else could you believe? Gather alternative information, different interpretations and new, more balanced or realistic beliefs that support your healing journey.

Embedding New Perspectives

Look for evidence that contradicts your original limiting beliefs around healing and supports your new alternatives. This could include success stories, scientific studies or personal experiences of healing and recovery. Develop positive affirmations and self-talk that counteract the negative beliefs.

Reinforcement and Repetition

New thoughts, when practised regularly, gradually replace old negative patterns, so repetition is key. Focus on regularly reinforcing your new empowering beliefs and replace self-limiting thoughts with more supportive and encouraging ones. Consciously bring this through on the emotional and physical level too, so you're not only thinking, but acting and feeling in alignment with these beliefs.

Congratulations! You've just completed the process known as cognitive restructuring. By addressing and releasing any thought-related blocks that are hindering your healing or desired future, you've unlocked the potential to do the same with your illness, your trauma and any other difficulty that's still lingering from the past.

Releasing the Past

Now you're ready to work specifically with the information revealed through connecting with the body and emotions. Again, we're gathering all the insights and information revealed through completing your timeline, alongside you *inner*-tuition, but this time you're processing these difficulties at the mental level of the Self.

We can start with finding what subconscious thoughts need to be addressed.

Uncovering Subconscious Thoughts

Take a moment to look at the table you created relating to the expression and lessons relayed to you through the language of the body (*page 175*).

Looking at those life lessons and the events from your timeline, reflect on what that situation you are carrying means about you. What beliefs are you left with? For example, if one of the memories that came up for you was that your partner left you for someone else, what have you decided that means about you, about others and about the world? Chances are that it is more to do with them than you, but it's likely that you've internalized some unhelpful, distorted or overgeneralized thinking.

Remember to express your thoughts and beliefs from the perspective of what *is*, rather than what *is not*. For example, in this scenario, rather than writing: 'I'm not wanted', you'd put down what you think you are; in this case: 'I am inferior'. To help, you can ask yourself, 'If I'm not wanted, then what am I?' This questioning enables you to come up with a direct statement that you can work with.

Uncovering Themes

What can be so detrimental here is using an identity statement, such as 'I am vulnerable'. Rather than that vulnerability relating specifically to how you felt in that one situation (i.e. 'I felt vulnerable when my partner left me'), you can internalize this as the truth about who you are. Watch out for this! If you carry this identity around in your subconscious mind as a general programme, it can become a lens through which you see the world, influencing how you perceive yourself in relation to other unrelated situations moving forwards. If this internalized inferiority is left unchecked, it can create the perfect conditions for external situations to emerge that reconfirm this new identity that you've amalgamated into the Self. That is, until you release it - which is exactly what we're going to do now!

When you've worked on a number of these issues, you might start to see some themes emerging, as there will be core beliefs and identities you are carrying subconsciously as a result. I have given a client example in the table below, so do take a look and then complete your own.

Choose an event or illness from the timeline	When I was seven years old and wet myself in front of the class because the teacher wouldn't let me go to the toilet.
Message speaking through the body and emotions	Severe psoriasis caused by my anger at the situation. The teacher got under my skin so my body created the 'thick skin' that I didn't have at the time. I needed to shed the shame, so my psoriasis caused my skin to come off. I also developed social anxiety and a panic disorder. This is manifesting the message that people are dangerous and that 'I would stay safe by keeping away!'
What does this situation or illness mean about me? 'I am...'	'I must have control over my body', 'I am an embarrassment'; 'People are cruel and going to hurt me'; 'I need to protect myself by staying away'; 'The world is unsafe'; 'I am vulnerable'.
What would I rather believe to be true about me now? 'I am...'	'I am strong and resilient'; 'I love and trust my body – it lets me experience life'; 'I create my own destiny'; 'I get to choose who to be around and where I want to go'; 'I am safe now'.
Plan of action to move forwards in a new way	I need to practise inner child work, keep challenging my belief system, future focus, visualizations of calming immune system, stress reduction techniques daily and join a local walking group.

I'm sure by now you can see that many of the beliefs you carry were formed in childhood or during difficult times, neither of which are likely to be relevant now, hence why they need releasing so they don't become the fuel for your future.

Once you've identified these negative thought patterns and identity statements, it's so important to generate what you would *rather* be true, so that this can be installed following the release of the old.

To process and release these negative thought patterns, you can go through the process of cognitive restructuring you employed earlier (*page 204*). EFT (*page 187*) and thymus tapping (*page 192*) are also great techniques for processing and releasing beliefs and thought energy.

To stay on top of your thoughts and thus your programming, it's important you learn to regularly shift from your reactive thinking mind into your observing mind, so you can become a passive observer of your thoughts. In doing so you can step back and watch your thinking, which will enable you to gain the awareness and inner wisdom needed to adapt and change if necessary. You do this in the same way you began sitting in the power (*page 72*), but rather than expanding out from the body and mind into the energy that surrounds you, you do so just with the mind. This enables you to become the presence behind the thoughts – that higher part of you that is aware that you're thinking.

We will utilize more of this observing mind in the next chapter, as in my opinion this is connected to the higher mind of the energy body. But before we move on to this, I will leave you with one last simple yet very effective technique for those unresolved memories you just can't shake off. Sometimes this is less about the details of the experience or the beliefs you carry, and more about how it's stored in the mind. If you're still getting emotionally triggered by a negatively charged memory that is replaying in your mind, then do this visualization:

Memory Re-coding

1. **Recall the memory**: Bring the negative memory to mind - what you saw, heard, felt, etc. - and rate the emotional intensity from 0-10.

2. **Notice how it's stored**: The chances are, if this memory is distressing you, you're fully immersed in it and are experiencing it *now* in just the same way as when it happened, which is why it's so distressing. You're back there, seeing it through your own eyes - you're the star of the movie.

3. **Separate yourself from the memory**: Become the observer of the movie in your mind; imagine you're sitting in the audience and see yourself in the scene.

4. **Switch the sub-modalities**: Now let's make it less vivid by turning off the sound, draining out the colour so it's black and white and changing it to a still photo in a frame, instead of a movie.

5. **Minimize the window**: Now, just as you might shut down an app on your phone, or close a programme on your computer that's been running in the background, you need to minimize the image. Just imagine pushing it away into the distance... further and further away, until it's just a black dot in the corner of the room.

6. **Check the intensity**: Bring the memory to mind once more and rate the emotional intensity again. What do you notice? How different does it seem now you've switched how it's stored in the filing cabinet of your mind?

Notice how this quick and easy mental reorganization of the memory instantly changes how you feel, along with the depth of those feelings, but notice also how your thoughts have shifted. I've had clients do this with some pretty horrific memories, then they leave bemused at how something so serious that has plagued them for years has literally lost its charge within a matter of minutes.

Usually one time is enough to discharge the energy from a memory and it will remain stored like this forever more. If on the off-chance that hasn't quite worked for you, though, that's perfectly fine. It happens! Just keep training your brain to shift the storage once again until it sticks!

CHAPTER 13

INNER-TUITION

Intuition is a complex phenomenon that is suggested by some theorists to be a purely neural process where the brain recognizes patterns and matches them to our past experiences.[1] There are also studies that focus on intuition as an energetic sensitivity in which the nervous system can detect information through electromagnetic fields in the environment,[2] such as in the sense of being stared at.[3] In addition to this, there are other theories that propose intuition to be linked to paranormal phenomena, such as precognition, telepathy and clairvoyance for example, suggesting connection and communication can exist beyond the constraints of time and space. A meta-analysis of nine studies of the paranormal, encompassing 1,000 participants, revealed statistically significant results in eight of the nine studies, proving that such phenomena is more than an anomaly.[4] Yet, in general, there is obviously still much debate regarding this topic amongst the scientific community. I personally believe that intuition is just another part of our sensory system that we're *all* capable of tuning in to and can all learn to develop.

I wonder what your experience of intuition is. Have you ever had a gut feeling about someone that turned out to be accurate?

Confusingly, I'd felt particularly protective towards my mother for the 24 hours prior to her fatal brain haemorrhage. I was uncharacteristically insistent on her resting, and on ensuring she look after herself and carry a mobile phone with her when taking Maya out in the pram. 'Who knows what might happen?' I remember saying. Not that there was anything *wrong* with her as such, nothing out of the ordinary for a lady in her 56th year. Yet an inner voice had been whispering to me. I knew I was picking up on something, but what was it? Why was I feeling so strange towards her? Something wasn't quite right, but I *just* couldn't quite grasp what was going on.

Even as those whispers became loud and indisputable, I still wasn't ready to piece together the puzzle. I'd been out visiting friends the previous evening and upon my return, all was eerily quiet and still – everyone was sleeping. As I crept through the hall, my attention was immediately caught by a framed photograph of my parents. Hanging across it, in a rather curious manner, was my mum's necklace – a gold crucifix. This was a very strange sight, as she never took it off, and would certainly never drape it over a photo.

No sooner had I noticed this perplexing placement than the voice came in loud and clear: 'That's how it will look when she's dead... That's how it will be tomorrow – when she's gone!' What kind of a thought was that? Who even thinks such a thing?

Accompanying this intrusion was a vision laid over my current view of reality. Nearly everything was identical, yet it also included my dad, who was in fact upstairs sleeping. In this vision he just sat there, perched on the edge of the armchair, forlorn, cradling his head in his hands – and in those few seconds all I could sense was grief.

I immediately brushed off this bizarre intrusion and went upstairs to snuggle up beside Maya. This was nothing more than nonsense. But sadly, nonsense, it was not.

Perhaps something like this has happened to you. You may yourself have denied a truth you weren't yet ready to see or able to compute. It's so easy to dismiss such unusual encounters as implausible and disregard our inner knowing as some foolish falsity. Then, when we've failed to take heed, the heavy 'what if' scolding comes in thick and fast, as we realize the signs were there all along. What if I'd stayed at home that morning? Perhaps she'd have recovered! At the very least, Maya wouldn't have been exposed to such a trauma unaided...

Or perhaps, just like 78 per cent of participants in a study by author and biologist Rupert Sheldrake, you're one of many people who experience 'telephone telepathy', when you think of someone who then unexpectedly calls.[5] Or maybe you've avoided a terrible accident because you just *knew* you needed to take a different route, or just 'by chance' missed your usual train. We all have the ability to *tune* in to our intuition, but when we're preoccupied by chatter at the level of the mind, consumed by the complaints of the physical body, or overwhelmed by emotion, any guidance from our higher Self gets stuck on mute. This is one of the reasons why I needed you to connect with all the other levels of Self before reconnecting with your intuition. I needed you to quieten the chatter, but I also wanted to show how it permeates *all* the levels, speaking through the body, the heart and the observing mind.

AN ENERGETIC IMPRINT

You need to be present and grounded in the sensing body to connect with your *inner*-tuition, which for the purpose of this book is defined as 'an instinctive knowing that emerges through our sensory perception rather than from conscious thought processing alone'.

I'm sure you've gathered by now that when I talk of 'sensory perception', I'm referring to our 'sixth' sense as well as the other five. It's through our physical senses that we interact and connect with the external world, but our intuition goes way beyond this. It's a form of intelligence that operates at a more highly attuned level of awareness, allowing us to access information and insights that aren't available to us through our physicality. I suppose the way in which I would describe this is that extra-sensory perception can access everything that the physical senses do, but rather than through the eyes, ears, mouth, skin and nose, this information consists of an energetic imprint available to us through the energy body.

If you remember, we have an energetic body or aura that surrounds and interpenetrates our physical body. Through sensing the energy between your hands (*page 65*) and sitting in the power (*page 72*), my hope is that you've now experienced this energy for yourself if you haven't done so before. This energy contains information about our physical, emotional, mental and spiritual wellbeing. By tuning in to our energy body through our *inner*-tuition, we can become more aware of the subtle energetic signals that are present and use this information to guide our actions, our decisions and our health. Thanks to the findings in quantum science, we know that our energy body is connected to all the other energetic realms in the Universe, so we can also tap into the unlimited potential within this consciousness for wisdom and guidance.

RECOGNIZING INTUITION

Through becoming more connected to your own *inner*-tuition, you can become more conscious of this energetic information. It's always been there as a line of communication, but your conscious awareness of it may have been lacking due to your past programming, belief systems or external distractions.

This information comes through to us from a higher-vibratory level of the Self. We can tell when we're receiving guidance from this space, as it has a different, more vibrant quality, and it kind of feels like it '*just is*'. It's a pure broadcast, untainted by the filter of our life experience or past programming.

As a result, there is no emotion, bias or judgement attached to it, which is why when needing guidance, it's ideal to connect with this level of intelligence and not go through the mind. The brain is a polarity organ, so it will often give you both sides of an argument, so as well as potentially clouding your judgement it can prompt thought processes that can keep you stuck in a loop of rumination.

Many people ask, 'How do I know if I'm hearing my own thoughts or hopeful wishes when seeking guidance?' In my experience, the key differentiator is that information that's self-generated will be likely to have some form of emotion attached to it and it often just reinforces something we already know to be true. On the other hand, guided information, whether from our *inner*-tuition, our higher Self, a spirit guide, angels, God or the Universe, is free from the influence of your conscious mind and so doesn't speak through your desires or expectations. This means the content can often be very direct and matter of fact, sometimes even surprising. At the same time, it can usually feel pretty understated, unemotional and impersonal, which is why it's so often disregarded or unheard. If we fail to take notice, however, it might well become persistent and repetitive until we do, whereas if it's coming from the mind, it's likely to soon move on to something new.

Intuition is often described as a 'gut feeling' or 'a sense of knowing that comes from within' and can manifest as an inner voice, a feeling of certainty or uncertainty, or a physical sensation. You can see below how each of our intuitive senses actually mirrors our physical ones:

- **Clairvoyance (clear seeing)**: The ability to see information beyond the physical senses, such as images, symbols or visions.

- **Clairaudience (clear hearing)**: The ability to hear information.

- **Clairsentience (clear feeling)**: The ability to feel information.

- **Claircognisance (clear knowing)**: The ability to know information.

- **Clairalience (clear smell):** The ability to smell information.

- **Clairgustance (clear taste):** The ability to taste information.

- **Clairtangency (clear touch):** The ability to receive information via touch.

RECONNECTING WITH YOUR INNER-TUITION

Now, I'm sure some of you reading this will have an awareness of a few of these senses already, and perhaps you regularly receive information from them, but for those of you who don't, they're not a 'gift' given to a select few, as many believe, they can be developed through training and practice. Yes, some people may be naturally more attuned, but that's the same with any sense or skill. Some people have a stronger sense of smell, others a good ear or precise vision, but as with everything, we all have our own individual strengths. It's likely, however, that you'll have an affinity for one of the 'clair senses' that mirrors your most dominant physical sense. For example, if you're a musician, then you'll most likely find clairaudience easier to develop; if you're very visual, then clairvoyance may be your thing; and if you're deeply empathic, then your clairsentience may be stronger.

For the purpose of reconnecting you with the level of your intuitive-Self and using it to help you process and release the pain from the past that resides in the present, we will focus on the main four senses, those that relate to clear seeing, hearing, feeling and knowing. This is because our intuitive abilities are primarily associated with the upper four chakras of the energy body: the crown, third eye, throat and heart (see opposite).

In order for your *inner*-tuition to flow freely, however, it's important to have a strong foundation in the lower chakras, as they play a crucial role in helping you to trust and feel secure in your intuitive abilities. A balanced root chakra, for instance, is essential for you to feel grounded and determines whether you feel a sense of safety and support when connecting with Source

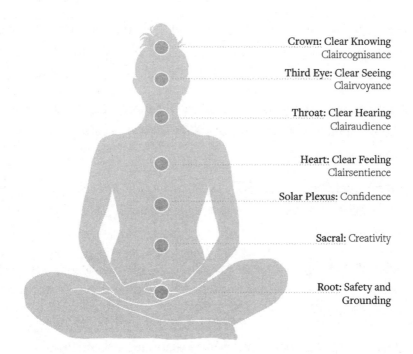

Crown: Clear Knowing
Claircognisance

Third Eye: Clear Seeing
Clairvoyance

Throat: Clear Hearing
Clairaudience

Heart: Clear Feeling
Clairsentience

Solar Plexus: Confidence

Sacral: Creativity

Root: Safety and
Grounding

The Chakras

energy. The sacral chakra affects your ability to access your creativity and self-expression, which, when balanced, enhances your ability to tap into your creative potential and manifest your desires. While the solar plexus chakra, which relates to your inner power, when balanced, can increase your confidence in trusting what comes from your *inner*-tuition, providing you with that 'gut feeling' you get about people and situations. So, balancing all seven chakras is vital to strengthening and expanding your intuition. When they are balanced and aligned, energy flows smoothly and body, heart, mind and spirit are all connected and working in harmony.

Chakra Sensing

As well as being connected to our intuition, our chakras hold the energy of those old stories, beliefs, habits and experiences from times past, and it has been suggested that each chakra is related to a particular stage of psychological and emotional development. See the list below for more information about these developmental stages. Do note, however, that the ages are just a guide, as everyone will follow their own specific timeline.

- **Root** (infancy, around 0–7 years old): Our earliest experiences, relating to our survival needs; our sense of safety, security, stability and basic trust

- **Sacral** (childhood, around 7–14 years old): Related to emotional development, creativity, sensuality and pleasure; it's a time when identity is first explored

- **Solar Plexus** (adolescence, around 14–21 years old): Related to our personal power, identity, willpower, confidence, self-worth and self-esteem

- **Heart** (early adulthood, around 21–28 years old): Related to relationships and our connection to others; love, compassion and empathy

- **Throat** (adulthood, around 28–35 years old): Related to communication and self-expression; finding our voice, creativity, authenticity and ability to express ourselves

- **Third Eye** (middle age, around 35–42 years old): Related to intuition, wisdom, insight and spiritual awareness

- **Crown** (late adulthood, around 42+ years old): Related to spiritual enlightenment and connection to higher consciousness, wisdom and transcendence.

This also means that if you're aware you're carrying a particular event from the past, it's important to check out what's happening with that chakra – is it blocked, over-active, under-active, misaligned or underdeveloped, for example?

It can be really helpful to connect the awareness you've gained about your present-past programming and conditioning with the knowledge from your energy body and chakra system. For example, you may suffer from a chronic digestive complaint and experience social anxiety, and upon joining the dots realize it goes back to being humiliated at your 18th birthday party when you couldn't stomach the feelings associated with your alcoholic father being drunk and rowdy. When looking at the chakra system, these physical symptoms make sense, as developmentally that age connects to the solar plexus, which relates to the health of the digestive system and is also related to confidence, self-worth and self-esteem. It could therefore be suggested that the energy in this chakra has been compromised, so we would need to check in to see, and focus on healing that area and the associated difficulties in order to prevent the manifestation of disease in the parts of the body in close proximity.

Knowing that each of your chakras holds your energetic history can really help to make sense of some of the difficulties you carry, along with any corresponding health and life issues. Take a look at the list on the previous page and cross-reference the difficulties you have been working on with the relevant developmental stage and the corresponding chakra to gain more insight into your life experience. At what age or developmental stage did the event, trauma or illness occur, and what aspect of the Self is it related to? Do your limiting beliefs or issues relate to a particular chakra or developmental stage, for example? What about your physical illnesses or your personal or relational lessons? Perhaps reflect on whether there is more insight and understanding to be gained here.

The chakras could be the very piece of the puzzle that provides you with further insight and supports your healing at an energetic level. So let's connect with them one by one and experience them for ourselves:

Connecting with the Chakras

Setting the Intention

At this stage, set your intention to simply connect with and sense your chakras. If you have already built up a connection, then use this exercise to gain the insight and wisdom needed in relation to the problems you've been working with.

Connecting with the Physical

Find yourself a comfortable space, drop into the body and allow your eyes to close off to the outside world. Focusing your awareness on the breath, connect to the body and begin a body scan (see page 44). What do you notice? What's present right now? Note any areas that feel tense, blocked or imbalanced, as these may correspond to the locations of the chakras.

Connecting with the Energy Body

Expand your awareness and focus on becoming attuned to the subtle energy within and around the body.

Now imagine a shimmering white ball of light above your head, its energy filling up the body with each and every breath. Allow that energy to flow down through the central core of the body, and visualize it flowing out through the soles of the feet, down roots reaching deep into the Earth.

Feeling grounded and connected, imagine drawing up energy from a similar ball of white light in the centre of the Earth. Draw it up into the body on the inhale and imagine the body and your energy body filling up with the frequency of this healing white light.

Connecting with the Chakras

Visualize each chakra in its respective location (see page 217) along the spine. Start with the root chakra at the base of the spine and move upwards, focusing on one chakra at a time. Don't worry if you can't see or feel the chakras, your intention will be enough. I like to imagine each chakra as a flower.

I open the petals when I want to activate the chakras, spin the energy clockwise and imagine breathing its essence into my whole body as if it's a mist. Do whatever works for you, but know that simply stating your intention will be enough for you to connect with and open your chakras.

Chakra Communication

Each time you open a chakra, scan through the body and send out the intention that you're safe and open to receiving the wisdom held within the body at that level, across all space and time.

Connect with the frequency of each chakra and remain open to any sensations in the body, alongside any thoughts, insights, feelings or emotions that arise. You may experience warmth, tingling, pressure or other subtle energetic sensations in the corresponding area. Bring in some mindfulness and just notice what comes through.

Intuitive Insights

Trust your intuition and any insights that come to you during the process. You may receive intuitive messages or information related to the state of each chakra or any energetic imbalances through any of the *clair* senses. If you're new to this, build trust, as it may not happen straight away.

Journalling

Open your journal, write down your experiences and reflect on what information came through – thoughts, images, memories, sensations, feelings, inner chatter, songs… This can provide insight, help you track your progress and deepen your understanding of your energy centres over time.

Closing Down

Once you feel ready, take a moment to return to the body and the breath. Go through the chakras one by one, from top to bottom, gently allowing the flowers to close, closing down the energy coming in from above your head and pulling up your roots. You could visualize zipping yourself up in a pastel pink sleeping bag, nice and snug.

Healing Visualizations

If there's a particular issue or illness you're working with then you can bring it to mind once you have opened the chakras so you can use a healing visualization. For example, when healing my pituitary tumours, I imagined the tumour as a block of ice (the fear) and gently melted it away with a beam of love, then sent in an army of Pac-Men (yes, I was a child of the eighties) to gobble up all the prolactin in my bloodstream and in my mind's eye created a gauge to watch the levels coming down. Whilst my pituitary gland was being soothed by an indigo energy (indigo for the third eye chakra), I continued with the visualization until all looked and felt well, and then in my mind I took myself to the moment when I would feel elation at seeing the test results showing the tumour had gone – and eventually it went! Interestingly, a mental representation of the immune system doing its job has actually been shown to aid the immune system,[6] so do keep an open mind about the power of visualizations. They may seem simple, but they *actually* work!

Whatever you're working on, bring in all your senses and see the outcome playing out just as you would like it to. It doesn't need to be related to your physical body; you can bring in healing visualizations to resolve anything – be creative! Do this once you've aligned all your chakras, but if you're aware of the issue being related to one in particular, be sure to imagine going into that chakra, filling yourself with its frequency and then completing the visualization from there.

Chakra Tapping

The process of chakra tapping involves gently tapping or massaging each chakra point to restore balance and harmony within body, heart, mind and soul.

This is another very quick and easy way to generate healing, process difficulties and release any blockages or disturbances in the flow of energy through the chakras and their corresponding physical organs.

For this, we're going to use a very similar process to the Emotional Freedom Technique (*page 187*), but instead of a set tapping sequence along the meridians, we will be tapping on the chakra points instead.

As each chakra is supposed to correspond to specific physical, emotional and spiritual aspect of our being, when working on healing and clearing them, we're again using a strategy to help us generate a fully Connected Self on all the levels.

Here are the directions for chakra tapping:

Chakra Tapping

1. Complete the usual preparation steps to feel centred and calm.

2. As with EFT, create a two-part set-up statement and use it three times with the karate chop point.

3. Now simply tap on each of the chakra points in the following order: root, sacral, solar plexus, heart, throat, third eye and crown, using your fingertips to tap or press gently on the area, and talk about the difficulty, issue, illness or belief you wish to clear. Whatever you're working with, remember to include how it affects your behaviour, the sensations in the body, your emotions, thoughts and beliefs. Spend a few moments at each point, tapping or massaging gently before moving on to the next.

4. When it's time to end, do another set of tapping whilst bringing your attention to the specific qualities and functions associated with each chakra. Visualize the energy flowing freely through it, bringing balance and harmony to that aspect of your being.

Heart-centred Consciousness

Another way to access your *inner*-tuition is through dropping into heart consciousness, through shifting into heart and brain coherence (harmony), which research has shown to improve intuition.[7] Until recently, the prevailing belief amongst psychologists was that your thoughts dictated your emotions, the assumption being that by working to alter your thought processes, you could then regulate your emotions. However, research in neuroscience has now revealed that intuition and emotional reactions actually happen much more quickly than cognitive processes,[8] meaning that it's your emotions and intuition that are most likely to be influencing your decisions and actions and not reasoning at the level of thought.

There is even evidence to suggest that the heart is involved in the processing and decoding of intuitive information, and in turn communicates this to the brain even *before* an adverse event occurs.[9,10] The same studies suggest that the heart is connected to a field of consciousness not bound by the classical limits of time and space, and that when we are in a coherent state, we are significantly more attuned to the information from the heart and thus better able to access intuitive guidance. There is also evidence to suggest that not only is the heart a key carrier of emotional information, it also provides electromagnetic communication between *people*, suggested to be similar to radio waves.[11] It is feasible to suggest, therefore, that it is through the energy of the heart that we access our intuition, which is a useful guide when trying to develop it.

CONNECTING WITH YOUR HIGHER SELF

We've already connected with the language of the body, emotions and thinking mind, and now it's time to bridge the gap between what I've been calling our *inner*-tuition, where we gain knowledge through the lower-vibrational levels of the Self that relate to this three-dimensional plane, and our intuition, where we're now focusing on receiving information from the consciousness of our higher Self. You could think of this as being from the heart chakra upwards.

Accessing Your Higher Self and Beyond

To connect with some inner guidance, here's my six-step process for accessing your higher Self and beyond (*see below*).

Ensure your external and internal environment are conducive to doing this work, and then begin sitting in the power of your energy body (*page 72*) before following the steps below:

1. **Define the problem**: Keep the conscious mind focused on what problem or issues you would like some guidance on. Acknowledge any beliefs and underlying emotions, along with how it feels in the body.

2. **Shift into the energy body**: Complete the process from Chapter 4 (*page 72*), so you can shift into the energy body and the observing mind through the experience of sitting in the power.

3. **Enhance heart and brain coherence**: Place your hands on your heart with the intention of bringing in a higher frequency. Remind yourself of something you're grateful for/someone you deeply love. Imagine breathing in and out through an open heart chakra, with a warm green or pink energy radiating out from it.

4. **Awaken the observing Self**: Now focus on your third eye chakra whilst also continuing to channel this higher frequency through the heart. Expand your awareness out from the thinking mind and into the observing mind.

5. **Connect with your higher Self**: Now it's time to imagine opening the crown chakra and inviting your higher Self to merge with your energy by speaking this intention in your mind. You may see an image, sense a presence, hear a voice – just know that they are connected and awaiting instruction.

6. **Asking for guidance**: Now you have an open channel, bring to mind the problem you were wishing to gain clarity with. You can approach this by asking the question in your mind/out loud and observing any change or insight that comes, or by asking a yes/no question to your heart directly.

What did you become aware of when calling in your higher Self? Be sure to detail the characteristics in your journal to help you spot it more quickly next time and build a sense of what it's like.

This is certainly a practice to do regularly as well as when you need specific guidance or support. It's the foundation for receiving any form of information from the psychic realms, so if you're also wanting to experiment with the possibility of accessing psychic communication, a useful expansion to this exercise is to follow steps 2–6 but then imagine a clear whiteboard in your mind's eye and invite your higher Self or spirit guides to communicate with you through this blank slate. Remember, this information can come through any of your senses, not just via vision. Just ask a question and wait for a response. Remain patient, as it takes regular practice; you're between two realms and need to train yourself to perceive what's already there – a bit like those magic eye images from the nineties that required a relaxed shift of gaze for you to capture the 3D image. In the same way, you may well be surprised the first time you truly experience some psychical phenomena!

Perhaps you can now see through your own experience that whilst we have a physical body, that physical body exists at a higher-vibrational frequency as an energy body, and whilst we have a thinking mind, that mind also exists on a higher-vibrational frequency as the observing mind and the higher mind. That higher mind is plugged into the collective consciousness and is streaming knowledge directly from Source, rather than through our life experience, conditioning and programming.

So when we listen through our heart consciousness, which connects into our emotional centre, and bring in the higher mind and the energy body, we're connected to the ability to heal ourselves. Although, we can't usually access those higher levels of consciousness needed for healing whilst we're still stuck in the lower vibrations of the physical body. Raising our vibration is key here.

CONNECTING WITH YOUR INTUITION

This book has been carefully curated to take you on a journey that has lessons simultaneously embedded in multiple dimensions with multiple intentions. The body scan, sitting in the power, visualizations and the mindfulness exercises, for example, help in the physical realm but were all introduced to prepare you for connecting with your intuition.

Before you can register and distinguish what information is coming from your higher Self, or even from other spiritual beings or levels of consciousness, you must first know yourself – how it feels to be you in your body, both physically and emotionally, what your inner voice sounds like in your mind, and what your energy body feels like. Then you can become aware of how different it feels when you've raised your vibration and are communicating with yourself from this space. It's also an important awareness to have if you're embarking on the next stage of the journey and choose to connect with other souls – whether they inhabit a body or not! You need to know who you are first, before you can have a *real* awareness of and connection with another person.

So, strengthening your intuitive connection won't solely come from the suggestions in this chapter, but from consistent practice of the various exercises you have already gathered in your toolbox. These exercises not only help maintain your connection at all levels of the Self, ensuring a clear channel and stable grounding, but also create the space for information to drop in. Along the way, you'll develop your senses and interpretation skills, enabling you to decipher the information given more effectively.

We live in a busy world, however, so if I was going to suggest one thing to do without fail, it would be the mindfulness and meditation exercises with the incorporation of the energy body. These are particularly useful when developing your intuition, as it's through the natural shift in brainwaves that we're able to establish a connection with our higher Self. Daily practice will not only benefit your mental and physical health, it will also bring a deeper awareness of the body, emotions and thoughts without attachment or judgement, thus opening space for intuitive information to flow in also.

In addition, consistently incorporating visualization into this practice of presence can help with enhancing intuition, as it enables you to consciously *exercise* your creative inner canvas. Journeying within the mind to create these visualizations and develop this skill is key, as this is where your clairvoyance is projected. Your intuitive-Self imprints images and movies in the same way – I could be looking at you right now in the physical realm, and yet at the same time connect with images at the level of my energy body through my third eye. Visualization exercises help you to further develop and interpret this. The word 'interpret' is key here, as sometimes the information given can be symbolic, which is another reason why you've been developing an alternative way of thinking, such as when we looked at the language of the body, for example.

So we really have established that various aspects of your being, including the body, thoughts, feelings, relationships and even life circumstances, are all speaking to you and providing valuable lessons for your personal growth and to enhance your health and wellbeing. Even your dreams can serve as a rich source of information.

Having become aware of, learnt and released these lessons, we're now going to shift away from the automatic input generated by past conditioning and consciously create new programming at each level of your being, by consciously connecting with and developing your future-Self.

CHAPTER 14

CONNECTING WITH YOUR FUTURE-SELF

Yay! This is it! You've made it to the moment where you could actually be at the beginning of a totally new chapter in your life! Having programmed a peaceful present and processed a painful past, it's here you get to leave that cocoon of change, spread your wings and take flight towards the limitless opportunities that await you in the new reality of your choosing.

This final stage of the process is where you'll connect with your future-Self timeline to embed your future-Self programming in the present, consciously calling this new reality into your life.

In the very first chapter of this book, you constructed a future-Self. Take a moment to reflect on that by reviewing your answers to the journal prompts (*page 27*). What are your thoughts on them now? What would you add to or change (if anything) about that potential future-Self? Are you still the same person who constructed that Self, or are you already becoming someone new?

Also check back over the other journal entries you've created whilst working through this book . What new perspectives have you integrated into your life and what have you let go of as a result?

Take some time to acknowledge all you have done to honour and nurture your whole Self and to congratulate yourself for having committed to doing the work. I congratulate you also for having a mind open enough to embrace the knowledge and skills required to access a new reality – one where you can leave your suffering and setbacks behind. But most of all, it's time to come back to the Self, to where and who you are in *this* moment, and to embrace that fully and with compassion, even if you've not yet engaged with or committed to doing the work.

THE CYCLE OF CHANGE

Change can be tough! It's not easy to break free from the deeply ingrained patterns that have shaped our lives, so it's common to feel a whole mix of emotions, including fear, doubt and uncertainty – even apathy! Creating a new version of yourself involves consciously and consistently making new choices in alignment with the 'future you' you are seeking and that can be challenging! *Lasting* change is rarely a simple process, as we often swiftly revert back to the known, but research has now identified a key journey that, with commitment and resilience, can lead to a new sustainable outcome.[1]

I wonder where you are in this cycle of change right now. Take a look at the diagram opposite and see what you think:

1. First, there is *pre-contemplation*, when someone is not ready, or unwilling, to consider change, or even unaware of the possibility. This may have been you before picking up this book, when perhaps you weren't even aware of any issues or desire for change in your life.

2. Secondly, there is *contemplation*, where someone is considering change, but hasn't yet acted. This is perhaps when you realize there's more to life, desire change or need to address a problem, but are reluctant to do anything about it or don't know how.

3. Thirdly, there is the *preparation* stage, when someone is preparing to make a move but isn't yet ready. Here you might be reading this book, but maybe your goals aren't yet in alignment with the change process, so you're not doing the exercises, you're just taking them all in as an observer right now.

4. Lastly, there's *action*, when the person is actively involved in change. This is when you're fully engaged in the process, value the outcome and are consciously changing and reviewing your choices in line with your future-Self.

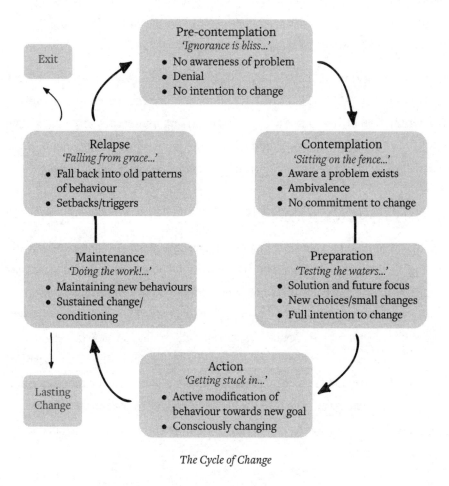

The Cycle of Change

This model reveals that people are often unwilling or resistant to change during the early stages. Knowing this may help you prepare for moving into a more proactive and committed phase. The diagram on the previous page illustrates this process.

Change may or may not come easily for you, but knowing these stages may help you to understand where you're at and find ways to stay on track and remain motivated, especially when you're feeling discouraged or have stopped believing in yourself.

What's good about this model is that it builds in maintenance and relapse as an inevitable part of the process, reinforcing change as a *feedback cycle* where we may take the lessons learnt and begin again.

You'll see that once the cycle of change is complete, you'll exit the process at 'lasting change'. This is equally valid when mastering a habit, recovering from addiction or living the life of your choosing, but it can only occur once you've maintained your new behaviours, which may occur after one cycle but will most likely be after beginning the process over and over again.

MAINTAINING CHANGE

Maintaining change can be challenging enough when you're actively ready to engage with the process, but if any part of you isn't fully invested, for whatever reason, such conflicts may undermine the process and set you up for a relapse. Including this as an expected part of a *cyclical* process of change will help you to see it as a feedback event from which you can learn, rather than fail. This perspective can help prevent you from abandoning the process of change when you face setbacks. It brings with it a level of self-acceptance and compassion, making change more achievable and more sustainable for you, so do remember this as you move forwards – there is no failure, only feedback!

Checking in:

When you've attempted to implement change in the past, where have you habitually come unstuck? Make a note of this. Such knowledge is helpful as you move forwards, so you can organize additional support.

Which of the stages in the Cycle of Change do you think you're in right now? Do you need support already? If so, make a plan. Go easy on yourself, though, and know you're exactly where you need to be to learn and grow.

How ready *are* you to begin living as your future-Self (0–100 per cent)? What needs to happen to shift that percentage higher?

For you to 'succeed' in whatever changes you wish to make in your life, you'll need to be conscious of these three important elements and work through them:

1. **Readiness to Change:** Do you have the resources, knowledge and ability to make lasting change happen? Is this something that you really want?

2. **Barriers to Change:** Is there anything preventing you from changing? What could get in the way? Is now the right time for you? Does anything else need to happen first?

3. **Likelihood of Relapse:** What might sabotage your plans for change or trigger a return to a former behaviour/life? How can you prevent this from happening/come back from relapse if it were to occur? What do you need to stay on track?

You'd think most people would seek professional help because they were motivated to make changes, but I'm still so surprised by the number of people commencing therapy at the request of someone else, or even to influence someone else to change. Either way, you can't force anything on anyone else – the only person you can change is yourself! But the truth is that you need much more than tools, knowledge and support to make change happen: you need to be personally invested in the change process and able to identify with and desire the end result – you need to find your *why*!

Finding Your Why

The comfort of familiarity so often keeps us anchored to the known and tethered to our past-Self, even if it no longer serves our highest good. This is why it so often takes the upheaval of those detrimental life events to redefine our narrative and to unearth the keys that unlock our liberation. Have you found this in your own life? That you hold on to relationships, behaviours or circumstances you know cause harm, yet instead of making the changes necessary to bring improvement, you just push forwards, fooling yourself you can weather the storm – that is, until you can't!

I know this was certainly the case for me. Even after all the traumas, illnesses and betrayal, I was still locked onto the misery of my old life with the precision of a missile heading for its target. I didn't want to be defined by my past, yet in reality I woke to it each and every day. So busy looking after everyone and everything else, I made no space for myself. That was, until I had nothing left to give! It took drowning in a secret depression and sinking to the depths of darkness for me to acknowledge I was slipping down a slope that led to the dead-end that was suicidal ideation.

To the outside world it was business as usual, but behind the daily mask I was crushed by the weight of my present pain, unable to envisage a brighter future beyond the next opportunity to switch off reality and escape into the solace of sleep. I'd hit rock bottom and was devoid of all life, yet with no option of ending it all, I was even more trapped. There was no way I could leave my two daughters... and therein came my *why*!

We all need a *why*, a reason for being, for getting up in the morning, for keeping ourselves alive. My daughters were mine. I was all they had, and I knew I could never inflict this suffering on them. In that lightbulb moment,

I came back to my purpose: 'to help people to help and heal themselves, and to do no harm unto others'. I felt I had no choice but to carry on with my life, yet I eventually realized that within that lack of choice I *did* have a choice – I could choose to carry on in pain, or I could carry on with purpose. Giving the latter option a chance, I vowed to dream with my eyes open instead of escaping to the safety of slumber. It was time to become someone new, so I energetically birthed her into existence in the way I will show you here. It was literally do or die!

To gain a distance and promote perspective, I did something completely out of character (and, to be honest, completely outside my price range): I spontaneously booked to go on a retreat in the Maldives. I needed to change environments to bring in the space where I could connect with all my levels of Self once more. On those beautiful islands, I raised my vibration, processed my pain and said goodbye to living as my present-past Self. I stepped onto a new timeline – the one with the *future me* writing this book – *et voilà*, here I am!

Embracing change doesn't mean leaving behind who you are, it means honouring your essence whilst embodying the possibility of who you can become. It's of paramount importance, therefore, to decide on exactly who that future-Self is and embrace them in the now! But just so you know, you don't need to fly to the Maldives to be with yourself enough to facilitate change – unless that's a part of your journey to becoming your future-Self, as it was with me.

So, let's begin by connecting you to your own *why*, to help clarify what your ideal future-Self will consist of and to consciously generate a more meaningful and intentional life. We can do this by looking at what values you hold and connecting with your purpose. Through this awareness you can make conscious choices that are in alignment with these values and aspirations. This will help you to create the sense of direction and clarity needed to move towards greater fulfilment, satisfaction, health and happiness.

THE JOURNEY WITHIN

Future-Self Values

Whether you've thought about them or not, your values are deeply held beliefs that shape your behaviour and decisions. Examples include honesty, compassion, fairness, integrity and freedom.

It's increasingly suggested in psychology that identifying, understanding and living in accordance with our core values is important for positive mental health and wellness. Whilst we can live a more fulfilled life when in alignment with our values, negative consequences arise when we don't. We become incongruent, inauthentic and thus much more likely to escape into bad habits, regress into childish or addictive behaviours, and have elevated stress levels, so our physical and mental health suffer.

We've already discussed how our cluttered and stressful lives are often spent running on autopilot, with life happening to us, rather than emanating from us. A by-product of this is we often become disconnected from our core values and focus more on living in alignment with the assumptions we've made about the values and expectations placed upon us by others, consuming 'stories' about what we 'should' value and falling deeper into the trap of creating a false Self.

Values are different for each and every person and can change over time according to our life experience. For this reason, we must regularly check that we're living in accordance with what matters most in the now. From this place, we get to construct goals that align with our current values, which in turn helps create a personally meaningful and fulfilling future.

In this instance we will be looking ahead to the beliefs, values and aspirations of the future-Self you wish to call into your life, so you can live according to them in the now. So step into that future-Self and embody them in your imagination before you begin the work. Your values now, as someone who's unwell, overweight and inactive, for example, will be very different from those of a future-Self who has run a marathon, eats 'clean' food and works as a health coach.

Don't worry if you aren't yet aware of the life you want for your future-Self, just embody how you want to *feel* as that future-Self. The following exercises will help connect you with the details.

Remember, our values inform our goals, but they're not the same. Put crudely, goals can be 'achieved', whereas values are more like a compass pointing us in the right direction. For example, you might have the goal of getting your children to school on time each day, which, for you, might sit within the value of 'being a good parent', which then resides within the core value of 'love'. So if we are to construct a future-Self that's compelling for you, it's important to identify your current values in relation to specific life domains and then set your goals accordingly.

Your Current and Future Values

Reflecting on Your Current Values

Reflect on what values you've been living in accordance with up to now. Where have they come from? When were they created? Who were you perhaps trying to please by living according to them – parent, teacher, friend, partner, boss? How might your life be if you took the power back and consciously lived according to your *own* values and just allowed them to flow through your life?

Uncovering Your Future Values

Take a look at the value domains below. Sit with each one, reflect on the questions, then see what thoughts and feelings surface. These will help you to connect with the values you hold in each area of your life so you can start to notice regular themes.

Always keep in mind the questions: 'What makes this important for me? What does it give me?' This helps you to unravel the layers to reveal your main purpose or your *why*. Remember, there are no 'right' answers, just what would make for a more meaningful life for *you*!

▲ **Self**: What personal qualities/traits do you value most? What personal achievements/accomplishments make you proud? What are your dreams/ aspirations? What lights you up?

▲ **Family**: What kind of relationship do you want to have with your family? What sort of child/sibling/grandchild/parent/grandparent do you want to be? What's your priority?

▲ **Intimate relationships**: What kind of spouse/partner do you want to be in a relationship? What kind of relationship do you want to be a part of? What sort of partnership do you want to build?

▲ **Parenting**: What sort of parent do you want to be? What qualities do you want your children to see in you? What kind of relationships do you want to build with them?

▲ **Social life/friendships**: What sort of friend do you want to be? How would you act? What kind of friendships are most important to cultivate? What kind of social life matters to you?

▲ **Health/wellbeing**: What kind of values do you have regarding your physical/mental health and wellbeing? How important is your health? What are your priorities? How would you look after yourself?

▲ **Recreation/fun/leisure**: How would you like to enjoy yourself? What relaxes you? When are you most playful? What location would that be in? Would that include anyone else? Who would that be?

▲ **Career/employment**: What kind of work matters to you? What qualities do you want to bring as an employee/boss? What kind of work relationships would you like to build?

▲ **Personal development**: How would you like to grow as a person? What kind of skills would you like to develop? What matters to you in education and learning? What would you like to know more about?

▲ **Citizenship/community**: What kind of environment do you want to be a part of? How do you want to contribute to your community? What kind of citizen would you like to be? How do you want to contribute?

▲ **Spirituality**: What do you see as your purpose for being? What kind of relationship do you want with God/nature/the Universe/the Earth? What brings you a sense of awe/perspective?

You'll now have a much clearer understanding of what you consider most valuable. This will form the foundation for how you live as your future-Self in the now.

Why not create your own table relating to each of these domains and write your current values in one column, then in the next, write from the perspective of your desired future-Self? If the two are vastly different and you've not been honouring your values in your life, this may bring some great insight into what's behind your current difficulties.

Now, we have just used our conscious mind to select our values, but when using the thinking mind alone we can unwittingly make choices based on what 'seems' better. For this reason we must also assess *intuitively* what values instinctively *feel* right to us, through consciously connecting with our higher Self.

Connecting with Core Values

Take the main values that showed up and ask yourself:

▲ 'How would embodying that value make me feel?'

▲ 'If I had that in my life, what would it give me?'

▲ 'What would [insert previous response] give me? How would I feel about that?'

Dig down through the levels until you identify what it is you really want from life, for example, love, peace, freedom, safety or connection.

///

This may take a little perseverance – for example, the core value of freedom might encompass top-level values of wellness, money, travel, education and self-expression.

Perhaps draw a spidergram with one of your core values in the middle and the supporting values and goals emanating from it. In practical terms, this provides you with a map of how to live in accordance with that core value.

See an alternative to this in the diagram below:

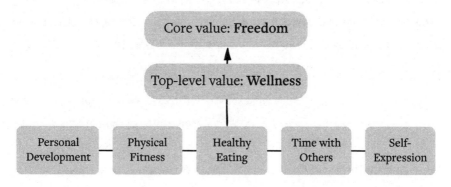

Example of Goals that Underpin Values

You can see from the diagram that there are numerous goals and values that feed into the top-level value of wellness, which then feeds into the core value of freedom. Here's a little tip to help differentiate what's what:

Clarifying Your Core Values

Quieten your mind and connect with the body, heart and energy body to allow the language of intuition to come through.

Bring your values to mind.

What do you feel?

Emotion is the key here. It's also the key to bringing your core values into your life. You can't *feel* wellness, nor can you *feel* personal development or physical fitness, not really, but if I were to ask you to close your eyes and *feel* freedom, *feel* love, *feel* peace, your bodily response would be on a whole new level, would it not? This is how you recognize a core value you need to live by.

If your values are the compass directing your life's journey, it's your emotions that generate the fuel that will get you there. This will remain unchanging, although the route can look different as your life changes over time.

Consider practical ways to create a *felt* sense of your core values in your life. Remember, they *must* be tailored to you!

Repeat these steps with each of your core values to help you to see what specific elements your future-Self will need to have in order for you to generate a fulfilled life.

///

The truth is, for you to make changes at the deepest level of your soul, you'll need to 'unbecome' the identity that has already been created and conditioned at the level of the material world. This is why we incorporated strategies to process and release you from your past in the previous chapter. Now we must fill up your levels one by one as we re-programme you for a favourable future.

EMBRACING YOUR PURPOSE

Aligning your actions with your values is essential if you're to experience a greater sense of fulfilment and authenticity in your life, as your values provide a compass for decision-making and guide you towards choices that are in harmony with your core beliefs.

Ikigai

A Japanese concept called *Ikigai*, roughly translating to 'reason for being', helps us to discover our sense of purpose and also encourages an alignment between our actions and what we truly value and find meaningful. In the context of *Ikigai*, identifying and living in accordance with your values is an essential part of discovering your purpose and experiencing a joyful life.

Often depicted as a Venn diagram (see opposite), *Ikigai* represents the intersection of four fundamental elements: what you love, what you're good at, what the world needs, and what you can be rewarded for.

If you're uncertain of your life purpose and don't know where you want your life to go, follow these six steps to explore your own *Ikigai*:

1. **Reflect on what you love:** Identify activities, hobbies or interests that bring you joy and make you feel alive. Consider the things that energize you and give you a sense of fulfilment.

2. **Assess what you're good at:** Recognize your unique skills, talents and strengths. Reflect on activities where you excel or receive positive feedback. These abilities can be both natural talents and developed skills.

3. **Consider what the world needs:** Explore the needs, problems or challenges in your community or society, or even globally. Think about how your skills and passions can contribute to addressing those needs or making a positive impact.

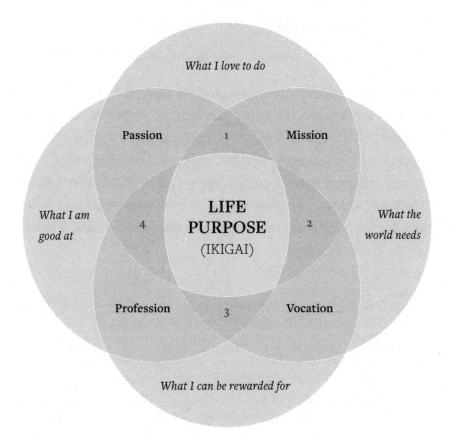

Venn diagram of Ikigai

4. **Identify what you can be rewarded for**: Consider the areas where you can potentially receive recognition, financial stability, or other forms of reward for your contributions.

5. **Look for the overlap**: Examine the intersections of what you love, what you're good at, what the world needs, and what you can be rewarded for. Seek the sweet spot where these elements converge, indicating your potential *Ikigai*.

6. **Experiment and refine**: Explore different avenues and activities that align with your identified *Ikigai*. Experiment with different combinations

to find the most fulfilling and rewarding pursuits. Refine your understanding of your *Ikigai* as you gain more insight and experience.

In essence, constructing your *Ikigai* involves aligning activities with your values to bring you joy, fulfil your potential, contribute to the needs of others, and find reward. By engaging in this process, you'll not only discover your purpose, you'll also add to the road map for your future-Self to live by. It can empower you to consciously construct a life that embodies your deepest aspirations, allowing you to live authentically and with a profound sense of meaning, unlocking your true potential and cultivating a purpose-driven existence.

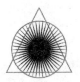

CHAPTER 15

YOUR FREEDOM FLIGHT –
EMBRACING A NEW REALITY!

Armed with the information and insights you've gained from the journey so far, you can now generate a plan that details the direction you would like your life to take. Whether it's a healthy lifestyle, a thriving business or a contented, loving relationship, now you've released the past and become conscious of what aligns with your future, you have a clean slate to begin re-programming the new.

RE-PROGRAMMING

To embark on the final stage of the Release and Re-programming Method, we need to expand our conscious awareness to a new level of being, unencumbered by past problems, difficulties or environments. It's from this vantage point – a place of higher vibration and awareness – that we can facilitate lasting change!

Now you have been incorporating strategies to turn down the stress-response system, and have processed and released some of the past programming that was fuelling it at a subconscious level, you're more able to access those higher-vibrational frequencies necessary to call in what you wish to manifest.

Stepping into Your Future

So let's map out the steps to get there. Follow the steps below and consider each detail in relation to the levels of Self. Remember to write in the present tense, for example 'I am...', and ensure it encompasses your *why*, helps to fulfil your greater purpose, is in alignment with your values and is within your control or power to make it happen.

Note how you *feel* as your future-Self, what beliefs you hold in order to live that way, what actions you take, what knowledge you have, what relationships you nurture. Let's really bring this future-Self to life!

1. **Clarify your vision**: Get clear on who you want to be. Reflect on your values, passions and aspirations. Define the qualities, achievements and experiences that align with your future-Self. Write down your vision and revisit it regularly – create a vision board and place it in clear sight (perhaps even on your phone).

2. **Set meaningful goals**: Break down your vision into tangible goals for each level of the Self. Make sure that your goals are specific, measurable, achievable, relevant and time-bound (SMART). Set both short-term and long-term goals to provide a clear road map for your journey.

3. **Develop an action plan**: Create a detailed action plan that addresses each level of the Self. Identify the steps and habits required. Break each goal into smaller, manageable tasks. Prioritize based on importance and develop a timeline for completion. Review regularly.

4. **Cultivate empowering habits**: Intentionally cultivate positive habits that align with your goals and vision for each dimension of the Self. Identify habits that support your future-Self and action

them daily. Use habit stacking to ensure they become conditioned and effortless.

5. **Seek supportive influences**: Surround yourself with people who share your values and aspirations. Have relationships that foster growth and accountability in all areas of Self. Connect with mentors, coaches or groups providing guidance/inspiration.

6. **Take action and persist**: Put a plan into action and commit to your journey. Take consistent steps to achieve goals across all levels of the Self, even when faced with obstacles/setbacks. Be resilient, persevere and celebrate each milestone achieved. Remember: There is no failure, only feedback!

7. **Reflect and adjust**: Regularly assess progress and reflect on how aligned your actions are with your future-Self vision. Revisit and revise goals, action plans and habits as needed. Stay adaptable and adjust for growth. Seek synergy amongst the different levels of the Self.

8. **Be in the present moment**: Keep a clear vision and close connection with your future-Self. Live this in the present moment, making decisions and choosing actions in alignment with your future-Self. Do three things that take you closer to your future-Self each day. Be it now!

TRANSFORMING TIMELINES: CONSCIOUSLY CALLING IN A NEW FUTURE-SELF

There's a future version of you living the life you've always dreamed of. This ideal future-Self is the result of all the efforts you're putting in right now. Remember, you've *always* held the power to shape that future in line with your utmost desires and can do so right now – starting from this very moment.

It's now time to send a powerful signal back to the present from that future-Self. This signal serves as a new blueprint, containing the revised coordinates that will guide you straight back towards your new desired future. Now, there may still be obstacles and events that will knock you off-track along the way – that's to be expected. But, armed with the strategies in this book, you now know you can get back up, reset your path and begin again!

One of the many psychic abilities that have accompanied me throughout my life is my ability to see down timelines and capture a future outcome that will occur should certain decisions take place.

For this book I have deconstructed this process and adapted the experience to create an exercise that will help you to consciously construct a potential future of your choosing, place it on your timeline, and become the person who can meet it there. So, are you ready? Let's begin.

Becoming Your Future-Self

Relax in a quiet spot for 30 minutes and follow these steps.

1. **Connect with your higher Self**: Connect with your breath and set the intention of transforming your timeline and reprogramming your future-Self. Elevate to heart consciousness and spend time sitting in the power. Call in your higher Self for guidance and remain open to *inner*-tuition from the levels of the Self.

2. **Generate your future-Self**: Visualize your desired future-Self at a point where what you want has already happened. Step into the movie and fully immerse yourself. Replay it repeatedly with all the senses and really *feel* the emotions before zooming out to be the observer of your timeline.

3. **Embed a new future-Self on your timeline**: Float above this future and release a golden ball of light representing this event. Witness

the timeline changing. Travel back to the present, dropping in new pivotal events and moments to readjust the timeline and trajectory of your present-Self. Zoom out to see your timeline as part of a vast network of possibilities, as one illuminated branch of life on the tree of possibility, energized from the roots.

4. **Expand the Timeline of Transformation**: Bring your timeline back online so it runs through you with the future ahead and past behind. Stretch it out towards future generations yet to be birthed and future lives you're yet to live. Observe these future scenarios playing down your timeline like movies on a TV screen.

5. **Physically connect with your future-Self**: Take a deep breath, open your eyes and carry the knowledge that you've set an intentional pathway to the future. To complete the final stage of transforming your timeline at the mental and physical level, write a letter from your new future-Self to yourself in the now (see below), and intentionally live each day with this future in mind.

You can also listen to an extended audio version of this exercise. You'll find it on my site (*page xxvi*) and in the audiobook.

Future-Self Letter

Now, having generated this new future-Self and cemented it energetically into your timeline, let's take this one step further and write a letter *from that* future-Self to the present-Self in the now. An example can be found on my website (*page xxvi*), but there's no right or wrong way to do this, just use your creativity.

1. Follow the previous steps to expand your new timeline and connect with your future-Self.

2. Write a letter to your present-Self from this place of future wisdom, having achieved all you've wished for.

3. Use the present tense and describe your achievements, offer insight and encourage growth.

4. Provide practical tips for overcoming challenges and express gratitude towards the present-Self for never giving up.

5. Give hints of great achievements to come, expressing pride and love towards your present-Self. Talk as if this were your most precious friend and imbue this letter with love.

6. Now imagine sending this letter down the timeline to be received by the you in the now.

7. Then switch back to the present-Self, read the letter, receive its wisdom and journal your responses.

This is simply another tool that sets reference points for you to find along your journey, and primes the body, mind and heart for what's coming next. This familiarity will bring a feeling of safety to times of change, preventing your fear response from getting in the way.

Be sure to really feel the positive emotions of this future-Self life, drawing it to you in the now through the energetic magnet that is your heart.

As we come to a close in these final moments of our journey, there's one level of the Self that needs further attention for this future-Self to be made manifest, and this is pivotal! Within the physical realm, you have looked at the future-Self from the perspective of the thinking *mind*, ensuring your values, beliefs and goals are in alignment with it, you've connected *emotionally* with the experience and felt it within the *body*, but this must also translate into *action*.

You now need to behave as your future-Self in the now to remain in alignment with the coordinates you have set. So be sure to consciously incorporate these habits into your daily living:

- **Present Focus:** Set your intention for how you want your day to play out from start to finish, taking note of how you wish to feel and what goals you need to achieve, specifically how that will practically factor into your day.

- **Future Focus:** Establish three things for tomorrow that will take you one step closer to your future-Self. Write them down and check them off the following night for accountability and reinforcement. Remember: the subconscious needs repetition to re-programme you to this future, so you'll need to reinforce it and take committed daily action!

- **Review:** Constantly review your goals and adjust them according to your present circumstances. Write them in a journal or visualize them through a vision board. By focusing on them before you go to sleep, your subconscious can work on any solutions you might need when you wake up – just ask for guidance.

- **Gratitude:** Habitually connect with the energy of gratitude for what you have in your life to programme abundance. Extend this to your future-Self. If you're grateful for this future in the now, the brain will act as if it's already happened, strengthening the probability that it will.

- **Subliminal Programming:** Sleep is the perfect state to absorb new suggestions. You need to be in a Theta brainwave state, reached via meditation/hypnosis. Ideally play a hypnosis track that's been personalized for you, but you can also use a more general meditation encompassing what you wish to install. Even replaying the track from this chapter will be of help.

- **Daily Check-in:** Whenever making decisions or actions, however big or small, get into the habit of asking yourself, 'Is this taking me closer to or further away from my future-Self?' If the answer is no, then be sure to make adjustments accordingly.

FINAL THOUGHTS

Congratulations! You've made it!

What an *amazing* journey you've been on to get here!

You've bravely travelled your timeline, connecting all the threads of unconscious programming from before, during and after your birth. Equipped with the teachings, tools and guidance from these chapters, you then uncovered, unravelled and unburdened yourself from this past, leaving you free to wear a new present-day reality, woven from a future-Self identity of your choosing.

Now that you've reached the end of this transformative experience and embraced this new reality – one that encompasses consciously living as a *multi*-dimensional being – take a moment to pause and reflect on the profound insights you've gained and the significant changes you've set in motion as a result. Consider how you feel now, knowing that you have unlimited possibility available to you, that you can be your own best healer, and that despite what difficulties come your way, you can continue to keep generating a life you love to live.

But remember, this book is just the beginning. *The Psychic Psychologist* has served as your guide, but the journey is ultimately yours to continue. You now possess the knowledge and ability to apply my Hierarchy of Healing protocol, so can maintain and reclaim an optimal level of health and wellness for the present, and for your future. You're also free to engage with the Release and Re-programming Method as and when you choose. So, when faced with more adversity, or if you've faltered and veered off course, you can relinquish what no longer fits, raise your vibrational frequency and switch to an alternate future-Self programming that aligns with your new vision. With the clarity of an awakened and fully connected body, heart, mind and spirit, you can always rediscover the Self you were destined to become.

Now it's time to congratulate yourself on having committed to doing the work, and for having a mind open enough to apply the knowledge and skills required to leave your suffering and setbacks behind. It's time to acknowledge all that you are and all that you've done to honour and nurture your *whole* authentic Self across the full expanse of your timeline. Having shifted its trajectory towards a future liberated from your past conditioning, your trauma, and your ancestral and past-life wounds, it's time to rejoice at having finally found freedom; at having healed from your past, found peace in the present and transformed your future.

So, let's embrace the wisdom of your inner tutor and the strength of your spirit, and remain open to listening to the language of your life as it speaks your truth through the physical, emotional, mental and spiritual Self.

This book began with facing the death of what once was and now, full circle, we find ourselves addressing another ending – or perhaps this marks a new beginning, for they are one and the same. So, I'd like to thank you for accompanying me on this journey, this quest to rebirth a fully connected and authentic Self. Now, as you venture forth, always remember that this future is set by you. So be the author of your own life, the healer of your own heart, and remain conscious for the next chapters of your life – they are yours to write.

It's time to dream with your eyes open!

NOTES AND REFERENCES

Chapter 1: The Self

1. Klussman, K., *et al.* (2022), 'The Importance of Awareness, Acceptance, and Alignment with the Self: A Framework for Understanding Self-connection', *Europe's Journal of Psychology*, 18(1): 120–31.

2. Bohm, D. (1952), 'A Suggested Interpretation of the Quantum Theory in Terms of "Hidden" Variables (I)', *Physical Review*, 85(2): 166–79.

3. Bohm, D. (1952), 'A Suggested Interpretation of the Quantum Theory in Terms of "Hidden" Variables (II)', *Physical Review*, 85(2): 180–93.

4. Rutherford, E. (1911), 'The Scattering of α and β Particles by Matter and the Structure of the Atom', *Philosophical Magazine*, 21(4): 669–88.

5. Weiskrantz, L. (2002), *Blindsight: A Case Study and Implications*, Oxford: Clarendon Press.

6. WebMD Editorial Contributors (2022), 'Dissociative Identity Disorder (Multiple Personality Disorder)': www.webmd.com/mental-health/dissociative-identity-disorder-multiple-personality-disorder [Accessed 4 August 2023].

7. Mitchell, S. (1889), 'Mary Reynolds: A Case of Double Consciousness': resource. nlm.nih.gov/101483385 [Accessed 4 August 2023].

8. Braun, B.G. (1983), 'Psychophysiologic Phenomena in Multiple Personality and Hypnosis', *American Journal of Clinical Hypnosis*, 26(2): 124–37.

9. Putnam, F.W., *et al.* (1986), 'The Clinical Phenomenology of Multiple Personality Disorder: A Review of 100 Recent Cases', *Journal of Clinical Psychiatry*, 47(6): 285–93.

10. Coons, P.M. (1980), 'Multiple Personality: Diagnostic Considerations', *Journal of Clinical Psychiatry*, 41(10): 330–36.

11. Taylor, W., and Martin, M. (1944), 'Multiple Personality', *Journal of Abnormal and Social Psychology*, 39(3): 281–300.

12. Goleman, D. (1988), 'Probing the Enigma of Multiple Personality', *The New York Times*, 28 June.

13. Pert, C. (2004), *Your Body is Your Subconscious Mind*, Louisville, CO: Sounds True.

14. Birnbaum, M.H., and Thomann, K. (1996), 'Visual Function in Multiple Personality Disorder', *Journal of the American Optometric Association*, 67(6): 327–34.

15. Strasburger, H., and Waldvogel, B. (2015), 'Sight and Blindness in the Same Person: Gating in the Visual System', *PsyCh*, 4(4): 178–85.

16. Page, S. J., *et al.* (2007), 'Mental Practice in Chronic Stroke', *Stroke*, 38(4): 1,293–7.

17. Kho, A.Y., *et al.* (2013), 'Meta-analysis on the Effect of Mental Imagery on Motor Recovery of the Hemiplegic Upper Extremity Function', *Australian Occupational Therapy Journal*, 61(2): 38–48.

18. Butler, A.J., and Page, S.J. (2006), 'Mental Practice with Motor Imagery: Evidence for Motor Recovery and Cortical Reorganization after Stroke', *Archives of Physical Medicine and Rehabilitation*, 87(12): 2–11.

19. Ranganathan, V.K., *et al.* (2004), 'From Mental Power to Muscle Power – Gaining Strength by Using the Mind', *Neuropsychologia*, 42(7): 944–56.

20. Pascual-Leone, A., *et al.* (1995), 'Modulation of Muscle Responses Evoked by Transcranial Magnetic Stimulation during the Acquisition of New Fine Motor Skills', *Journal of Neurophysiology*, 74(3): 1,037–45.

21. Reddan, M.C., *et al.* (2018), 'Attenuating Neural Threat Expression with Imagination', *Neuron*, 100(4): 994–1,005.

Chapter 2: An Absence of Self – Mind, Body and Soul(less) Living

1. World Health Organization (2022), 'Noncommunicable Diseases': www.who.int/news-room/fact-sheets/detail/noncommunicable-diseases [Accessed 12 July 2023].

2. World Health Organization (2023), 'Depressive Disorder (Depression)': www.who.int/news-room/fact-sheets/detail/depression [Accessed 12 July 2023].

3. World Health Organization (2021), 'Suicide': www.who.int/news-room/fact-sheets/detail/suicide [Accessed 12 July 2023].

4. World Health Organization (2019), 'Suicide': www.who.int/health-topics/suicide [Accessed 12 July 2023].

5. Solomon, G.F. (2001), 'The Development and History of Psychoimmunology', *The Link between Religion and Health: Psychoneuroimmunology and the Faith Factor* (eds H.G. Koenig and H.J. Cohen), Oxford: Oxford University Press.

6. Pert, C.B., *et al.* (1985), 'Neuropeptides and Their Receptors: A Psychosomatic Network', *Journal of Immunology*, 135(2 Suppl): 820s–26s.

7. Solomon, *op. cit.*

8. Khoury, B., *et al.* (2013), 'Mindfulness-based Therapy: A Comprehensive Meta-analysis', *Clinical Psychology Review*, 33(6): 763–71.

9. Miller, L., *et al.* (2014), 'Neuroanatomical Correlates of Religiosity and Spirituality: A Study in Adults at High and Low Familial Risk for Depression', *JAMA Psychiatry*, 71(2): 128–35.

10. Stanley, E.A. (2019), *Widen the Window: Training Your Brain and Body to Thrive During Stress and Recover from Trauma*, New York: Avery.

11. MacLean, P.D. (1990), *The Triune Brain in Evolution: Role in Paleocerebral Functions*, New York; London: Plenum Press.

12. Steffen, P.R., *et al.* (2022), 'The Brain Is Adaptive, Not Triune: How the Brain Responds to Threat, Challenge, and Change', *Frontiers in Psychiatry*, 13.

13. Porges, S.W. (2001), 'The Polyvagal Theory: Phylogenetic Substrates of a Social Nervous System', *International Journal of Psychophysiology*, 42(2): 123–46.

14. Porges, S.W. (2011), *The Polyvagal Theory: Neurophysiological Foundations of Emotions, Attachment, Communication, and Self-regulation*, New York: Norton.

15. Cannon, W.B. (2017), *Bodily Changes in Pain, Hunger, Fear and Rage*, Andesite Press.

16. Carmody, J., and Baer, R.A. (2008), 'Relationships Between Mindfulness Practice and Levels of Mindfulness, Medical and Psychological Symptoms and Well-being in a Mindfulness-based Stress Reduction Program', *Journal of Behavioral Medicine*, 31(1): 23–33.

17. Lengacher, C.A., *et al.* (2009), 'Randomized Controlled Trial of Mindfulness-based Stress Reduction (MBSR) for Survivors of Breast Cancer', *Psycho-Oncology*, 18(12): 1,261–72.

18. Grossman, P., *et al.* (2004), 'Mindfulness-based Stress Reduction and Health Benefits: A Meta-Analysis', *Journal of Psychosomatic Research*, 57(1): 35-43.

19. Ditto, B., *et al.* (2006), 'Short-term Autonomic and Cardiovascular Effects of Mindfulness Body Scan Meditation', *Annals of Behavioral Medicine*, 32(3): 227–34.

Chapter 4: Wellness is an Inside Job

1. McManus, D.E. (2017), 'Reiki Is Better Than Placebo and Has Broad Potential as a Complementary Health Therapy', *Journal of Evidence-Based Complementary & Alternative Medicine*, 22(4): 1,051–7.

2. Zadro, S., and P. Stapleton (2022), 'Does Reiki Benefit Mental Health Symptoms Above Placebo?', *Frontiers in Psychology*, 13: 897312.

3. Demir Doğan, M. (2018), 'The Effect of Reiki on Pain: A Meta-analysis', *Complementary Therapies in Clinical Practice*, May 31: 384–7.

4. Billot, M., *et al.* (2019), 'Reiki Therapy for Pain, Anxiety and Quality of Life', *BMJ Supportive & Palliative Care*, 9(4): 434–38.

5. Olson, K., *et al.* (2003), 'A Phase II Trial of Reiki for the Management of Pain in Advanced Cancer Patients', *Journal of Pain and Symptom Management*, 26(5): 990–97.

6. Achterberg, J., *et al.* (2005), 'Evidence for Correlations Between Distant Intentionality and Brain Function in Recipients: A Functional Magnetic Resonance Imaging Analysis', *Journal of Alternative and Complementary Medicine*, 11(6): 965–71.

7. Standish, L.J., *et al.* (2003), 'Evidence of Correlated Functional Magnetic Resonance Imaging Signals between Distant Human Brains', *Alternative Therapies in Health and Medicine*, 9(1): 122–5, 128.

Chapter 5: The Release and Re-programming Method

1. Borkovec, T.D., *et al.* (1983), 'Stimulus Control Applications to the Treatment of Worry', *Behaviour Research and Therapy*, 21(3): 247–51.

2. McGowan, S.K., and Behar, E. (2012), 'A Preliminary Investigation of Stimulus Control Training for Worry', *Behavior Modification*, 37(1): 90–112.

3. Dugas, M.J., *et al.* (1998), 'Generalized Anxiety Disorder: A Preliminary Test of a Conceptual Model', *Behaviour Research and Therapy*, 36(2): 215–26.

4. Fincham, G.W., *et al.* (2023), 'Effect of Breathwork on Stress and Mental Health: A Meta-analysis of Randomised-Controlled Trials', *Scientific Reports*, 13(1).

5. Banushi, B., *et al.* (2023), 'Breathwork Interventions for Adults with Clinically Diagnosed Anxiety Disorders: A Scoping Review', *Brain Sciences*, 13(2): 256.

6. Descilo, T., *et al.* (2010), 'Effects of a Yoga Breath Intervention Alone and in Combination with an Exposure Therapy for Post-Traumatic Stress Disorder and Depression in Survivors of the 2004 South-East Asia Tsunami', *Acta Psychiatrica Scandinavica*, 121(4): 289–300.

7. Gerbarg, P.L., *et al.* (2019), 'Breath Practices for Survivor and Caregiver Stress, Depression, and Post-traumatic Stress Disorder: Connection, Co-regulation, Compassion', *OBM Integrative and Complementary Medicine*, 4(3):1–1.

8. Bhargava, R., *et al.* (1988), 'Autonomic Responses to Breath Holding and its Variations Following *Pranayama*', *Indian Journal of Physiology and Pharmacology*, 32(4): 257–64.

9. Zaccaro, A., *et al.* (2018), 'How Breath-Control Can Change Your Life: A Systematic Review on Psycho-Physiological Correlates of Slow Breathing', *Frontiers in Human Neuroscience*, 12(353).

10. Kabat-Zinn, J., and Hanh, T.N. (2013), *Full Catastrophe Living*, New York: Random House Publishing Group.

11. Creswell, J.D., *et al.* (2019), 'Mindfulness Training and Physical Health', *Psychosomatic Medicine*, 81(3): 224–32.

12. Bhattacharya, S., and Hofmann, S.G. (2023), 'Mindfulness-based Interventions for Anxiety and Depression', *Clinics in Integrated Care*, 16: 100138.

13. Khoury, B., *et al.* (2013), 'Mindfulness-based Therapy: A Comprehensive Meta-analysis', *Clinical Psychology Review*, 33(6): 763–71.

14. Goldberg, S.B., *et al.* (2018), 'Mindfulness-based Interventions for Psychiatric Disorders: A Systematic Review and Meta-analysis', *Clinical Psychology Review*, 59(59): 52–60.

15. Black, D.S., and Slavich, G.M. (2016), 'Mindfulness Meditation and the Immune System: A Systematic Review of Randomized Controlled Trials', *Annals of the New York Academy of Sciences*, 1373(1):13–24.

16. Creswell, J.D. (2017), 'Mindfulness Interventions', *Annual Review of Psychology*, 68(1): 491–516.

17. Doll, A., *et al.* (2016), 'Mindful Attention to Breath Regulates Emotions via Increased Amygdala–prefrontal Cortex Connectivity', *NeuroImage*, 134: 305–13.

18. Segal, Z.V., *et al.* (2018), *Mindfulness-based Cognitive Therapy for Depression*, 2nd ed., New York: The Guilford Press.

19. Mooventhan, A., and Nivethitha, L. (2014), 'Scientific Evidence-based Effects of Hydrotherapy on Various Systems of the Body', *North American Journal of Medical Sciences*, 6(5): 199.

20. Tipton, M.J., *et al.* (2017), 'Cold Water Immersion: Kill or Cure?', *Experimental Physiology*, 102(11): 1,335–55.

21. Shevchuk, N.A. (2008), 'Adapted Cold Shower as a Potential Treatment for Depression', *Medical Hypotheses*, 70(5): 995–1,001.

22. Shevchuk, N.A. (2007), 'Possible Use of Repeated Cold Stress for Reducing Fatigue in Chronic Fatigue Syndrome: A Hypothesis', *Behavioral and Brain Functions*, 3(1): 55.

23. Kujawski, S., *et al.* (2022), 'Combination of Whole Body Cryotherapy with Static Stretching Exercises Reduces Fatigue and Improves Functioning of the Autonomic Nervous System in Chronic Fatigue Syndrome', *Journal of Translational Medicine*, 20(1).

24. Wim Hof Method, 'What are the Benefits of Cold Therapy?': www.wimhofmethod.com/cold-therapy [Accessed 15 April 2023].

25. Ober, C. (2014), *Earthing: The Most Important Health Discovery Ever!*, Laguna Beach, CA: Basic Health Publications, Inc.

26. Chevalier, G., *et al.* (2012), 'Earthing: Health Implications of Reconnecting the Human Body to the Earth's Surface Electrons', *Journal of Environmental and Public Health*, 1–8.

27. Oschman, J., *et al.* (2015), 'The Effects of Grounding (Earthing) on Inflammation, the Immune Response, Wound Healing, and Prevention and Treatment of Chronic Inflammatory and Autoimmune Diseases', *Journal of Inflammation Research*, 8: 83.

28. Chevalier, G., *et al.* (2019), 'The Effects of Grounding (Earthing) on Bodyworkers' Pain and Overall Quality of Life: A Randomized Controlled Trial', *EXPLORE*, 15(3): 181–90.

29. Oschman, *op. cit.*

30. Chevalier (2019), *op. cit.*

31. Chevalier, G. (2015), 'The Effect of Grounding the Human Body on Mood', *Psychological Reports*, 116(2): 534–42.

32. Elkin, H.K., and Winter, A. (2018), 'Grounding Patients with Hypertension Improves Blood Pressure: A Case History Series Study', *Alternative Therapies in Health and Medicine*, 24(6): 46–50.

33. Toussaint, L., *et al.* (2021), 'Effectiveness of Progressive Muscle Relaxation, Deep Breathing, and Guided Imagery in Promoting Psychological and Physiological States of Relaxation', ed. R. Taylor-Piliae, *Evidence-Based Complementary and Alternative Medicine*, (1): 1–8.

34. Cohen, M., and Tyagi, A. (2016), 'Yoga and Heart Rate Variability: A Comprehensive Review of the Literature', *International Journal of Yoga*, 9(2): 97.

35. Field, T., *et al.* (2013), 'Tai Chi/Yoga Reduces Prenatal Depression, Anxiety and Sleep Disturbances', *Complementary Therapies in Clinical Practice*, 19(1): 6–10.

36. Streeter, C., *et al.* (2018), 'Effects of Yoga on Thalamic Gamma-Aminobutyric Acid, Mood and Depression: Analysis of Two Randomized Controlled Trials', *Journal of Neuropsychiatry*, 8(6): 1,923–39.

37. O'Shea, M., *et al.* (2022), 'Integration of Hatha Yoga and Evidence-based Psychological Treatments for Common Mental Disorders: An Evidence Map', *Journal of Clinical Psychology*, 78(9).

38. Field, T. (2016), 'Massage Therapy Research Review', *Complementary Therapies in Clinical Practice*, 24: 19–31.

39. Engen, D.J., *et al.* (2012), 'Feasibility and Effect of Chair Massage Offered to Nurses during Work Hours on Stress-related Symptoms: A Pilot Study', *Complementary Therapies in Clinical Practice*, (4): 212–15.

Chapter 6: Gaining an Awareness of Past Programming

1. Lee S. (2021), '*The Wisdom of Trauma – Dr. Gabor Maté*': drgabormate.com/the-wisdom-of-trauma/ [Accessed 10 August 2023].

Chapter 7: From Womb to World

1. Coussons-Read, M.E. (2013), 'Effects of Prenatal Stress on Pregnancy and Human Development: Mechanisms and Pathways', *Obstetric Medicine*, 6(2): 52–7.

2. Pearsall, P.P. (1999), *The Heart's Code*, London: Harmony Publishers

3. Gustafson, C., and Lipton, B. (2017), 'The Jump From Cell Culture to Consciousness', *Integrative Medicine*, 16(6): 44–50.

4. *Ibid.*

5. Lipton, B.H. (2006), *The Wisdom of Your Cells: How Your Beliefs Control Your Biology*, Louisville, CO: Sounds True, Inc.

6. Verny, T. and Weintraub, P., (2014), *Nurturing the Unborn Child: A Nine-Month Program for Soothing, Stimulating, and Communicating with Your Baby*, Open Road Media.

7. *Ibid.*

8. Coussons-Read, *op cit.*

9. O'Connor, T.G., *et al.* (2012), 'Prenatal Cortisol Exposure Predicts Infant Cortisol Response to Acute Stress', *Developmental Psychobiology*, 55(2): 145–55.

10. Wong, Y.J., *et al.* (2016), 'Does Gratitude Writing Improve the Mental Health of Psychotherapy Clients? Evidence from a Randomized Controlled Trial', *Psychotherapy Research*, 28(2): 192–202.

11. Cheng, S.T., *et al.* (2015), 'Improving Mental Health in Health Care Practitioners: Randomized Controlled Trial of a Gratitude Intervention', *Journal of Consulting and Clinical Psychology*, 83(1): 177–86.

12. Redwine, L.S., *et al.* (2016), 'Pilot Randomized Study of a Gratitude Journaling Intervention on Heart Rate Variability and Inflammatory Biomarkers in Patients with Stage B Heart Failure', *Psychosomatic Medicine*, 78(6): 667–76.

13. Emmons, R.A., and McCullough, M.E. (2003), 'Counting Blessings versus Burdens: An Experimental Investigation of Gratitude and Subjective Well-being in Daily Life', *Journal of Personality & Social Psychology*, 84(2): 377–89.

14. Felitti, V.J., *et al.* (1998), 'Relationship of Childhood Abuse and Household Dysfunction to Many of the Leading Causes of Death in Adults: The Adverse Childhood Experiences (ACE) Study', *American Journal of Preventive Medicine*, 14(4): 245–58.

15. Redwine, *op. cit.*

16. Centers for Disease Control and Prevention (2020), 'About the CDC-Kaiser ACE Study': www.cdc.gov/violenceprevention/aces/about.html [Accessed 4 August 2023].

Chapter 8: Awakening Your Ancestry

1. Gustafson, C. and Lipton, B. (2017), 'The Jump From Cell Culture to Consciousness', *Integrative medicine*, 16(6): 44–50.

2. Alegría-Torres, J.A., *et al.* (2011), 'Epigenetics and lifestyle', *Epigenomics* (3): 267–77.

3. Babar, Q., *et al.* (2022), 'Novel Epigenetic Therapeutic Strategies and Targets in Cancer', *Biochimica et Biophysica Acta Molecular Basis of Disease*, 1,868(12): 166–552.

4. Dawson, Mark A., and Kouzarides, T. (2012), 'Cancer Epigenetics: From Mechanism to Therapy', *Cell*, 150(1): 12–27.

5. Wang, G., *et al.* (2022), 'Epigenetics in Congenital Heart Disease', *Journal of the American Heart Association*, 11(7).

6. Lardenoije, R., *et al.* (2015), 'The Epigenetics of Aging and Neurodegeneration', *Progress in Neurobiology*, 131: 21–64.

7. McGowan, P.O., *et al.* (2009), 'Epigenetic regulation of the glucocorticoid receptor in human brain associates with childhood abuse', *Nature Neuroscience*, 12(3): 342–8.

8. Hacket, J. (2013), 'Scientists discover how epigenetic information could be inherited', University of Cambridge: www.cam.ac.uk/research/news/scientists-discover-how-epigenetic-information-could-be-inherited [Accessed 22 August 2023].

9. Dias, B.G. and Ressler, K.J. (2013), 'Parental olfactory experience influences behaviour and neural structure in subsequent generations', *Nature Neuroscience*, 17(1): 89–96.

10. Yehuda R., *et al.* (2016), 'Holocaust Exposure Induced Intergenerational Effects on FKBP5 Methylation', *Biological Psychiatry*, 80(5): 372–80.

11. Yehuda, R., *et al.* (2005), 'Transgenerational Effects of Posttraumatic Stress Disorder in Babies of Mothers Exposed to the World Trade Centre Attacks during Pregnancy', *The Journal of Clinical Endocrinology & Metabolism*, 90(7): 4115–8.

12. Yehuda, R. and Seckl, J. (2011), 'Minireview: Stress-Related Psychiatric Disorders with Low Cortisol Levels: A Metabolic Hypothesis', *Endocrinology*, 152(12): 4496–503.

13. Yehuda R., *et al.* (2000), 'Low Cortisol and Risk for PTSD in Adult Offspring of Holocaust Survivors'. *American Journal of Psychiatry*, 157(8): 1252–9.

14. Rodriguez, T., (2015), 'Descendants of Holocaust Survivors Have Altered Stress Hormones', *Scientific American Mind*, 26(2).

15. Bale, T.L. (2015), 'Epigenetic and transgenerational reprogramming of brain development', *Nature Reviews Neuroscience*, 16(6): 332–44.

16. Hales, C.N. and Barker, D.J. (2001), 'The thrifty phenotype hypothesis', *British Medical Bulletin*, 60(1): 5–20.

17. Franklin, T.B., *et al.* (2010), 'Epigenetic Transmission of the Impact of Early Stress Across Generations', *Biological Psychiatry*, 68(5): 408–15.

18. Weaver, I.C.G., *et al.* (2004), 'Epigenetic programming by maternal behaviour', *Nature Neuroscience*, 7(8): 847–54.

19. Dias, *op. cit.*

20. Lipton, B.H. (2016), *The Biology of Belief: Unleashing the Power of Consciousness, Matter & Miracles*, Carlsbad, California: Hay House, Inc.

21. Kaliman, P., *et al.* (2014), 'Rapid changes in histone deacetylases and inflammatory gene expression in expert meditators', *Psychoneuroendocrinology*, 40: 96–107.

22. Freedman, F., (2021), 'Maternal emotions and human development': birthlight. com/maternal-emotions-and-human-development [Accessed 22 August 2023].

Chapter 9: A Life before Life

1. Curcio, C.S.S., and Moreira-Almeida, A. (2018), 'Who Does Believe in Life After Death? Brazilian Data from Clinical and Non-clinical Samples', *Journal of Religion and Health*, 58(4): 1,217–34.

2. Stark, R., and Sims Bainbridge, W. (1996), *A Theory of Religion*, New Brunswick, NJ: Rutgers University Press.

3. World Values Survey (2022), WVS database: www.worldvaluessurvey.org/ WVSDocumentationWV7.jsp [Accessed 11 June 2022].

4. Tanne, J. H. (2007), 'Ian Pretyman Stevenson'. *BMJ*, 334 (7595): 700.

5. Tucker, J.B. (2008), 'Children's Reports of Past-Life Memories: A Review', *EXPLORE*, 4(4): 244–8.

6. Tucker, J.B., (2021), *Before*, New York: St. Martin's Essentials.

7. Lucchetti G., *et al.* (2013), 'Rare Medical Conditions and Suggestive Past-Life Memories: A Case Report and Literature Review.', *EXPLORE*, 9(6): 372–6.

8. Tucker, J.B. (2008), 'Ian Stevenson and Cases of the Reincarnation Type': med.virginia.edu/perceptual-studies/wp-content/uploads/sites/360/2016/12/ REI36Tucker-1.pdf [Accessed 11 June 2022].

9. Tanne, *op. cit.*

10. Weiss, B. (1994), *Many Lives, Many Masters*, London: Piatkus.

Chapter 10: Processing a Painful Past

1. Maslow, A.H. (1943), 'A Theory of Human Motivation', *Psychological Review*, 50(4): 370–96.

2. Maté, G. (2003), *When the Body Says No: The Cost of Hidden Stress*, London: Ebury Publishing.

3. Thomas, S.P., *et al.* (2000), 'Anger and Cancer: An Analysis of the Linkages', *Cancer Nursing*, 23(5): 344–9.

4. Rose, E. (2012), *Metaphysical Anatomy*, Vol. I, United States: Evette Rose.

5. Shapiro, D. (2012), *Your Body Speaks Your Mind*, London: Piatkus.

6. van der Kolk, B. (2015), *The Body Keeps the Score: Brain, Mind and Body in the Healing of Trauma*, London: Penguin.

7. Levine, P. (1997), *Waking the Tiger: The Innate Capacity to Transform Overwhelming Experiences*, Berkeley, CA: North Atlantic Books.

Chapter 11: Clearing Unprocessed Emotions

1. Pert, C.B. (1997), *Molecules of Emotion*, New York: Simon and Schuster.

2. Lieberman, M.D., *et al.* (2007), 'Putting feelings into words: affect labeling disrupts amygdala activity in response to affective stimuli', *Psychological Science*, 18(5): 421–8.

3. Nummenmaa, L., *et al.* (2013), 'Bodily maps of emotions', *PNAS*, 111(2).

4. Maté, G., (2011), *When the Body Says No*, Canada: Vintage.

5. Hawkins, D.R. (2015), *Healing and Recovery*, Carlsbad, California: Hay House, Inc.

6. *Ibid.*

7. Plutchik, R. (2001), 'The Nature of Emotions: Human emotions have deep evolutionary roots, a fact that may explain their complexity and provide tools for clinical practice', *American Scientist*, 89(4): 344–50.

8. Church, D., *et al.* (2022), 'Clinical EFT as an evidence-based practice for the treatment of psychological and physiological conditions: A systematic review', *Frontiers in Psychology*, 10(13).

9. Sebastian, B. and Nelms, J. (2017), 'The Effectiveness of Emotional Freedom Techniques in the Treatment of Posttraumatic Stress Disorder: A Meta-Analysis', *EXPLORE*, 13(1): 16–25.

10. National Institute for Health and Care Excellence Final Post-traumatic stress disorder [D] Evidence reviews for psychological, psychosocial and other non-pharmacological interventions for the treatment of PTSD in adults NICE guideline NG116 Evidence reviews, (2018): www.nice.org.uk/guidance/ng116/evidence/evidence-review-d-psychological-psychosocial-and-other-nonpharmacological-interventions-for-the-treatment-of-ptsd-in-adults-pdf-6602621008 [Accessed 30 October 2022].

Chapter 12: The Mind Matters

1. Tseng, J. and Poppenk, J. (2020), 'Brain meta-state transitions demarcate thoughts across task contexts exposing the mental noise of trait neuroticism', *Nature Communications*, 11(1): 3480.

2. Lipton, B.H. (2016), *The Biology of Belief: Unleashing the Power of Consciousness, Matter & Miracles*, Carlsbad, California: Hay House, Inc.

3. Pert, C.B. (1997), *Molecules of Emotion*, New York: Simon and Schuster.

4. Emoto, M. (2011), *The Hidden Messages in Water*, New York: Simon and Schuster.

5. Spinhoven, P., *et al.* (2018), 'Repetitive negative thinking as a predictor of depression and anxiety: A longitudinal cohort study', *Journal of Affective Disorders*, 241: 216–25.

6. Tennen, H. and Affleck, G. (1990), 'Blaming Others for Threatening Events', *Psychological Bulletin*, 108: 209–32.

7. Tyra, A.T., *et al.* (2020), 'Cynical hostility relates to a lack of habituation of the cardiovascular response to repeated acute stress', *Psychophysiology*, 57(12).

8. Sartorius, N. (2018), 'Depression and Diabetes', *Dialogues in Clinical Neuroscience*, 20(1): 47–52.

9. How Does Depression Affect the Heart?: www.heart.org/en/healthy-living/healthy-lifestyle/mental-health-and-wellbeing/how-does-depression-affect-the-heart [Accessed 23 August 2023].

10. Liu, Y.Z., *et al.* (2017), 'Inflammation: The Common Pathway of Stress-Related Diseases', *Frontiers in Human Neuroscience*, 11(316).

11. Walsh, S., *et al.* (2016), 'The Application of Positive Psychotherapy in Mental Health Care: A Systematic Review', *Journal of Clinical Psychology*, 73(6): 638–51.

12. Moser, J.S., *et al.* (2017), 'Third-person self-talk facilitates emotion regulation without engaging cognitive control: Converging evidence from ERP and fMRI', *Scientific Reports*, 7(1).

13. Hatzigeorgiadis, A., *et al.* (2011), 'Self-Talk and Sports Performance', *Perspectives on Psychological Science*, 6(4): 348–56.

14. Pietrowsky, R. and Mikutta, J. (2012), 'Effects of Positive Psychology Interventions in Depressive Patients—A Randomized Control Study', *Psychology*, 3(12): 1067–73.

15. Chakhssi, F., *et al.* (2018), 'The effect of positive psychology interventions on well-being and distress in clinical samples with psychiatric or somatic disorders: a systematic review and meta-analysis', *BMC Psychiatry*, 18(1).

16. Lipton, *op cit.*

17. Parker, G., *et al.* (2003), 'Clinical trials of antidepressant medications are producing meaningless results', *British Journal of Psychiatry*, 183(2): 102–4.

18. Barsky, A.J. (2022), 'Nonspecific Medication Side Effects and the Nocebo Phenomenon', *JAMA*, 287(5): 622.

19. Colloca, L. and Miller, F.G. (2011), 'The Nocebo Effect and Its Relevance for Clinical Practice', *Psychosomatic Medicine*, 73(7): 598–603.

20. Holder, D. (2008), 'Health: beware negative self-fulfilling prophecy': www.seattletimes.com/seattle-news/health/health-beware-negative-self-fulfilling-prophecy/ [Accessed 4 August 2023].

Chapter 13: *Inner-Tuition*

1. Hodgkinson, G.P., *et al.* (2008), 'Intuition: A fundamental bridging construct in the behavioural sciences', *British Journal of Psychology*, 99(1): 1–27.

2. Halberg, F., *et al.* (2011), 'Time Structures (Chronomes) Of The Blood Circulation, Populations, Health, Human Affairs And Space Weather, *World Heart Journal*, 3(1).

3. Sheldrake, R. (2013), *The Sense of Being Stared At*, New York: Simon and Schuster.

4. Bem, D.J. (2011), 'Feeling the future: experimental evidence for anomalous retroactive influences on cognition and affect', *Journal of Personality and Social Psychology*, 100(3): 407–25.

5. Sheldrake, R. (2001), 'The Anticipation of Telephone Calls: a Survey in California', *The Journal of Parapsychology*, 65: 145–56.

6. Hamilton, D.R. (2018), *How Your Mind Can Heal Your Body*, London: Hay House UK.

7. Mccraty R. and Zayas, M. (2014), 'Intuitive Intelligence, Self-regulation, and Lifting Consciousness', *Global Advances in Health and Medicine*, 3(2): 56–65.

8. LeDoux, J.E. (1996), *The Emotional Brain: The Mysterious Underpinnings of Emotional Life*, London: Phoenix.

9. McCraty, R., *et al.* (2004), 'Electrophysiological Evidence of Intuition: Part 1 The Surprising Role of the Heart', *The Journal of Alternative and Complementary Medicine*, 10(1): 133–43.

10. McCraty R., *et al.* (2004), 'Electrophysiological Evidence of Intuition: Part 2 A System-Wide Process?', *The Journal of Alternative and Complementary Medicine*, 10(2): 325–36.

11. McCraty, R. (2014), 'The Energetic Heart: Biolectromagnetic Interactions Within and Between People', *The Neuropsychotherapist*, 6(1): 22–43.

Chapter 14: Connecting with your Future-Self

1. Prochaska, J.O. and DiClemente, C.C. (1983), 'Stages and processes of self-change of smoking: Toward an integrative model of change', *Journal of Consulting and Clinical Psychology*, 51(3): 390–5.

ACKNOWLEDGEMENTS

I would firstly like to extend my gratitude to Hay House Inc. for hosting the Writer's Workshop as a route for new authors such as myself to showcase their work and submit a book proposal to win a publishing contract. In particular, my deepest thanks go out to everyone at Hay House UK that has provided the support to help bring this book to the world for all to read. Specifically to Michelle Pilley, Managing Director and Publisher of Hay House UK, for recognizing the potential in my manuscript and for entrusting me to deliver it – without her, this book simply would not exist. To my Commissioning Editor, Kezia Bayard-White, for all her support and faith along the way – I'm sure my last-minute 'pulling it out of the bag' had you needing your own therapy. To Lizzie Henry for her magic touch when editing, reducing and restructuring the original manuscript. To Rebecca Flynn, who worked her own magic also, stepping in as a last-minute editor and piecing the project together in a way that helped to keep things on track. To Jo Burgess and Katherine O'Brien who I know are about to work their magic with the book publicity and promotion. The design team, the typesetter and everyone else who has played a part in the moulding of this book, however big or small, I thank you all.

Thanks also to Jennifer Kubiak at KN Literary for her help and support with the book proposal that would eventually see me enter the Hay House Writer's Workshop competition and emerge as one of the grand prize winners. To

Jacq Burns, founder of The London Writers' Club, for her editorial support and for walking alongside me, supporting me as I emptied my soul onto the page. Thanks also to my amazing friend Claire Ralph for doing the same, and to Donna Louise Hay for her design input, support and cheerleading of The Psychic Psychologist brand and book.

A huge thank you to the wonderful Gordon Smith for being so kind and generous in agreeing to write the foreword to this book. I am so grateful for all your support over the years, for your teachings and for originally naming me as 'The Psychic Psychologist'. I may not have liked it at first, but I am certainly learning to embrace it now – I couldn't have done this without you!

Thank you to Mel Wells for encouraging me to take on this new identity of The Psychic Psychologist, despite my professional reservations – who'd have thought back then I'd become inspired to go on to also write a book published by Hay House. Thank you also to Shannon Kaiser and Jessica Huie MBE, for your invaluable enthusiasm and professional guidance along the way.

A big shout out to Maya, Lyla and Darren, for your unwavering belief in me and for tirelessly standing by my side, lifting me up during those times of doubt when it all got a bit too much – my love for you knows no bounds – thank you! I extend this love to so many other dear friends for their support and encouragement also – you know who you are. You've either had to listen to a book bore over the past two years or have waited patiently for me to emerge from my book writing hibernation – it's clearly time for a party!

I offer my utmost love and appreciation to all those clients who have kindly agreed to share some of their lives within these pages to help bring this work to life. Thank you all for this amazing gift. Thanks also to the rest of my clients who have allowed me the privilege of walking alongside them as they embarked on their own journeys of transformation. I have learnt so much from working with each and every one of you, so in many ways, you too have contributed to the wisdom I share within this book.

I must also give credit to the science. To those scientists and great minds who have worked tirelessly to provide the research that backs up the theories and exercises within this book and have allowed evidence-based practice to emerge within the field of psychology – your contribution is invaluable.

Finally, I thank you, the reader, for investing your time and energy in this book and for trusting that it would provide you with some of the ingredients you need to live a more fulfilling life. I thank you for giving me the opportunity to fulfil my own life purpose, which is to help you to help yourself and for being open-minded enough to embrace your whole authentic Self so you could 'do the work'. It's because of you this book was birthed, and it's because of you I found the strength to push through the procrastination and all those late nights and early mornings. So, thank you for standing by me and making this all worthwhile.

And to my mum, my dad and my brother, thank you for supporting and loving me from the other side – I hope I've done you proud!

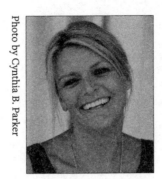

Photo by Cynthia B. Parker

About the Author

Amanda Charles, CPsychol, is a highly sought-after and experienced International Chartered Counselling Psychologist (BPS), Registered Practitioner Psychologist (HCPC), Life Coach, NLP Practitioner, Hypno-Psychotherapist, Reiki Healer, Psychic-Medium, and Meditation and Mindfulness Teacher.

Now branded as The Psychic Psychologist, Amanda has combined her two decades of extensive therapeutic experience with her exceptional intuitive and healing capabilities to formulate the Release and Re-programming Method. When used alongside her Hierarchy of Healing protocol, this methodology helps people to reconnect with others and their authentic selves, so that they can heal from their past and consciously generate a life they love to live.

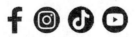

@thepsychicpsychologist

www.thepsychicpsychologist.com

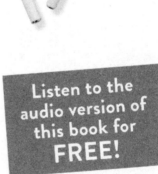
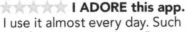

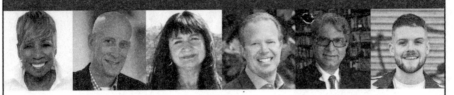

CONNECT WITH

HAY HOUSE

ONLINE

🌐 hayhouse.co.uk   **f** @hayhouse

📷 @hayhouseuk   𝕏 @hayhouseuk

▶ @hayhouseuk   ♪ @hayhouseuk

Find out all about our latest books & card decks • Be the first to know about exclusive discounts • Interact with our authors in live broadcasts • Celebrate the cycle of the seasons with us • Watch free videos from your favourite authors • Connect with like-minded souls

'The gateways to wisdom and knowledge are always open.'

Louise Hay